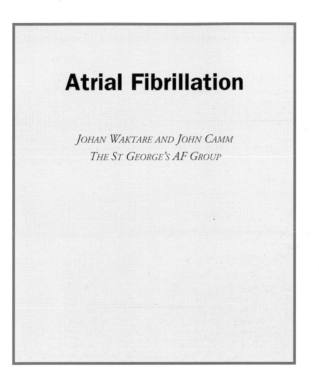

Atrial Fibrillation

Johan Waktare and John Camm
The St George's AF Group

MARTIN DUNITZ

Supported by an unrestricted educational grant from Pfizer Inc.

© Martin Dunitz 2000

First published in the United Kingdom
in 2000 by:

Martin Dunitz Ltd
The Livery House
7–9 Pratt Street
London NW1 0AE

A CIP record for this book is available from
the British Library.

ISBN 1-85317-715-6

Distributed in the USA, Canada and Brazil by:

Blackwell Science Inc
Commerce Place
350 Main Street
Malden
MA02148-5018
USA
Tel: 1-800-215-1000
Printed and bound in Italy

Contents

Acknowledgements

The authors would like to gratefully acknowledge the substantial contributions made by the St George's AF Group: Owen Obel, Mark Gallagher, Mark Sopher, Naab Al Saadi.
We are grateful for the assistance of Graham Leech, Mike Davies and Mandy Graham who helped with individual figures included in this book.

Preface

Atrial fibrillation is the most common tachyarrhythmia in the western world. As recently as the 1980s, it was the one arrhythmia most physicians thought they knew how to treat. The clinical standard was to do one's best to suppress atrial fibrillation with an antiarrhythmic agent, and to provide ventricular rate control during periods of atrial fibrillation. In the last 10–15 years, a good deal more has been learned about atrial fibrillation and its treatment. Much of it is helpful, and has changed our treatment regimens, but some of it has been rather confounding and worrisome. Epidemiological studies, physiological studies, and clinical trials have been at the forefront of providing us with what is new about atrial fibrillation and its treatment. Important new data are available concerning the association of atrial fibrillation with systemic embolism and stroke, the importance of warfarin therapy with an established therapeutic INR range, the importance and difficulty of ventricular rate control during atrial fibrillation, the association of tachycardia-mediated cardiomyopathy as a result of inadequate control of ventricular rate during atrial fibrillation, the role of devices in the treatment of atrial fibrillation, new concepts in cardioversion, new approaches to cure atrial fibrillation using surgical or catheter ablation techniques, and new attitudes towards drug therapy of atrial fibrillation. This handbook by Waktare and Camm covers all this and more in a compact but complete text that should help all clinicians who treat patients with atrial fibrillation. And the references supplied will provide avenues for more in-depth exploration of various subjects. In sum, this will be a handy reference that will get the reader to the core of what matters in a most practical and clinically satisfactory manner. It is a most helpful and welcome addition to the field.

Albert L Waldo, MD
The Walter H Pritchard Professor of Cardiology and
Professor of Medicine
Cleveland, OH

Foreword

Atrial fibrillation is so prevalent that almost every type of doctor has some responsibility for its diagnosis, investigation and treatment. Obviously the arrhythmologist, cardiologist and general physician are often required to formulate treatment strategies, but general practitioners are usually responsible for initial identification of patients and for supervision of their long-term care. Surgeons and anaesthetists must be wary of atrial fibrillation since it may complicate their surgery or anaesthetic. However, it is the physician dealing with the elderly who most frequently encounters this problem as it is often the product of age-related degeneration and disease. Its prevalence increases as the numbers of elderly people increase and it is predominantly in this group that atrial fibrillation wreaks its most serious adverse effects: heart failure and stroke.

This short text is intended for all those doctors and health professionals who deal with patients suffering from atrial fibrillation. The book attempts to present the modern approach to this arrhythmia that is no longer considered almost 'normal'. Since so much of atrial fibrillation can now be cured, very substantially suppressed or effectively controlled, those responsible for caring for patients with this condition must adopt an active and often an interventional approach to its management that is no longer a simple matter of a prescription for digoxin, and another appointment. Often the referral of the patient to a specialist physician or cardiologist should be considered.

We have attempted to keep the text short and to the point, and to illustrate the book freely. We hope that the result is readable and informative. We have included some important references to seminal and original research and to excellent reviews.

This short book is the product of the Atrial Fibrillation section in the Department of Cardiological Sciences at St George's Hospital Medical School, London. Those who contributed ideas, sections of text and illustrations were Johan Waktare, Owen Obel, Mark Gallagher, Mark Sopher, Naab Al Saadi and John Camm. The design and editing was by John Camm and Johan Waktare.

Johan Waktare and John Camm

Introduction

Atrial fibrillation has recently attracted considerable interest because it has finally been realized that it is not sufficiently benign to be regarded as an acceptable alternative to normal sinus rhythm.

Atrial fibrillation is commonplace (almost 1% of the population), provokes many symptoms (particularly, limited exercise tolerance and lethargy), is associated with considerable morbidity (heart failure, stroke, other arrhythmias) and mortality (predominantly cardiac or cerebrovascular) and causes a greatly impaired quality of life.

Some striking new strategies have emerged in recent years: in every patient it is now necessary to consider whether he/she can be cardioverted and maintained in sinus rhythm, anticoagulation is essential for very many patients with atrial fibrillation (or flutter), and if cardioversion is contemplated it should be undertaken as soon as possible to prevent atrial remodelling and the development of refractory atrial fibrillation.

A new range of therapies has now become available. Non-pharmacological approaches such as surgery, atrioventricular

(AV) ablation, pacemakers, atrioverters, etc. may be highly successful. New drugs have been developed or are close to becoming approved for use in atrial fibrillation, for example dofetilide, ibutilide and azimilide.

Atrial fibrillation is now managed more actively and more successfully. However, the long-term value of these new strategies and new treatments has yet to be established.

Key references

1. Waktare JEP, Camm AJ. Atrial fibrillation begets trouble. *Heart.* (1997) **77**: 393–4.

2. Falk RH, Podrid PJ. *Atrial Fibrillation: Mechanisms and Management.* (Raven Press, New York, 1997).

3. Murgatroyd FD, Camm AJ. *Non-Pharmacological Treatment of Atrial Fibrillation.* (Futura: Armonk, New York, 1997).

Epidemiology

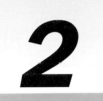

Incidence and prevalence

Atrial fibrillation (AF) is the most common sustained arrhythmia and accounts for more days in hospital than any other arrhythmia. The overall prevalence of AF in the general population is 0.5–1%, but the incidence of new AF rises sharply in old age, doubling with each decade of later life (Figure 1). In the Framingham study the biennial incidence

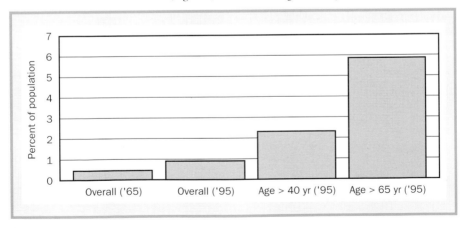

Figure 1
The prevalence of AF in 1965 (Ostrander et al. Circ (1965) 31: 888–98) and in 1995 (Feinberg et al. Arch Int Med (1995) 155: 469–73). The excess of AF in the elderly population is demonstrated by the 1995 study (70% of those with AF are over 65 years). Even after correcting for the age population distribution, the incidence of AF has risen over recent years.

(number of patients who developed AF over a 2-year period) rose from 0.6/1000 in those aged 55–64 years to 7.6/1000 in the 85–94-year age group. This striking association of AF with old age results in a prevalence of AF of more than 5% in those over the age of 65 years and more than 17% in octogenarians. Men are approximately 50% more likely to develop AF than women. However, since women survive for longer, about half of all patients with AF are female. The age independent prevalence of AF appears to be increasing, particularly in men. The reasons for this increase are not clear (it is not due to ascertainment bias) but may relate to improved survival, particularly after myocardial infarction or with heart failure. The incidence of paroxysmal AF is difficult to determine accurately since the arrhythmia may often be asymptomatic and its definition varies in many of the large studies. Thus, the reported incidence of paroxysmal AF varies from 25 to 62% of all cases of AF.

Causes and precipitants of AF

The clinical causes and precipitants of AF can be divided into cardiac (Table 1) and noncardiac (Table 2) factors. In a significant proportion of patients several such factors may be involved. The decreasing incidence of rheumatic heart disease in the developed world has led to the emergence of hypertension, ischaemic heart disease and heart failure as the leading clinical associations with AF.

AF usually occurs in conjunction with cardiovascular disease. Of the various cardiac risk factors, congestive cardiac failure is associated with the highest age-adjusted odds

Table 1
Cardiac causes and precipitants of AF.

> Congestive cardiac failure
> Valvular heart disease (especially mitral valve disease)
> Hypertension
> Myocardial infarction
> Pericarditis
> Myocarditis
> Congenital heart disease
> Hypertrophic cardiomyopathy
> Wolff–Parkinson–White syndrome
> Postcardiac surgery

Table 2
Noncardiac causes and precipitants of AF.

Thyrotoxicosis
Phaeochromocytoma
Electrolyte disturbances (particularly hypokalaemia)
Excessive alcohol consumption (binge-drinking and chronic, long-term use)
Recreational drug use (e.g. Cocaine, Ecstasy)
Acute and chronic pulmonary/pulmonary–vascular disease including:
Pneumonia
Acute pulmonary embolism
Chronic obstructive airways disease

ratio of developing AF. Valvular heart disease, hypertension and myocardial infarction are also strongly related to AF. There is a definite association with coronary artery disease, but it is complex. AF complicating the early course of myocardial infarction may be due to thrombotic occlusion or stenosis proximal to the sinus node artery and/or to atrial infarction, while AF in the setting of chronic angina is usually seen when there is left ventricular impairment, especially diastolic dysfunction, as a result of the ischaemic heart disease. There is no clear evidence that AF is associated with stable angina in the absence of infarction. The association of valvular heart disease and AF is more common in women with mitral valve disease. AF occurs in approximately 40% of patients with mitral stenosis and 75% of cases of significant mitral regurgitation. At one time atrial fibrillation

was known as 'the mitral pulse' particularly because of the association with mitral regurgitation. Other echocardiographic parameters which identify a higher risk of developing AF are given in Table 3.

AF may be caused by pericarditis, myocarditis and congenital heart disease, and is present in 5% of patients with hypertrophic cardiomyopathy. AF complicates the postoperative course of 25–30% of patients undergoing coronary artery bypass grafts and an even higher proportion of valvular procedures. AF is seen in association with sinus node disease in the sick sinus syndrome, often comprising the tachycardia component of the 'tachy-brady' syndrome. In 10–30% of patients with Wolff–Parkinson–White (WPW) syndrome AF occurs at some stage, and may be potentially life threatening (see

Table 3
Echocardiographic parameters associated with increased risk of AF.

Left atrial enlargement
Left ventricular systolic dysfunction
Left ventricular hypertrophy, or diastolic dysfunction from another cause
Valvular abnormalities
Mitral stenosis (usually due to rheumatic heart disease)
Mitral regurgitation (with mitral annular calcification > valve prolapse)
Severe aortic valve disease (through effect on left ventricle)
Congenital heart disease
Typically occurs late, preceded by more organized arrhythmias such as atrial flutter
Post-surgical/post-'correction'

Table 4
Risk factors for postoperative AF.

Cardiac surgery > thoracic surgery > nonthoracic major surgery
In cardiac surgery: valvular > nonvalvular
Prior history of AF
Increased duration of signal averaged P wave
Left ventricular systolic dysfunction
Advanced age
Preoperative withdrawal of beta blockers

Chapter 9). AF may also result from the 'degeneration' of AV nodal re-entrant tachycardia, atrial flutter or atrial tachycardia (the 'tachycardia-on-tachycardia' phenomenon).

Several noncardiac factors may cause or contribute to the development of AF. These include thyrotoxicosis, electrolyte disturbances (particularly hypokalaemia), and excessive alcohol consumption. Acute and chronic pulmonary or pulmonary–vascular disease such as pneumonia, acute pulmonary embolism, and chronic obstructive airways disease may present with AF. The relationship between AF and the degree and pattern of alcohol consumption is yet to be fully defined. While the Framingham study did not suggest a relationship between alcohol consumption and AF, several studies have shown that brief periods of heavy intake (binge drinking) can precipitate acute AF. Intermittently high alcohol intake can precipitate recurrent AF (the 'holiday heart'), and may increase the likelihood of AF recurrence after successful cardioversion. Long-term alcohol use is associated with a higher incidence and more frequent recurrence of AF, and alcoholic cardiomyopathy often comprises AF and myocardial dysfunction.

Given the above plethora of structural abnormalities and noncardiac diseases associated with AF, the possible role of genetic factors had not been considered until recently. However a large Spanish family with members who developed AF without other associated disease and at a young age has been reported.

The gene was localized to the long arm of chromosome 10, but has not as yet been identified. However the same site appeared implicated in two subsequent families. A genetic basis for the disorder was proven in these families, and many other cases are now being evaluated. It seems unlikely that familial factors will prove to be the major factor in most cases of AF, but a genetic predisposition may prove the determining factor to explain why only a proportion of those with, for example, severe mitral valve disease develop AF.

The prevalence of AF occurring in the absence of any detectable cardiac disease ('lone or idiopathic AF') amounts to around 10% of cases of permanent AF, but up to half of all paroxysmal AF (Figure 2). However, the precise proportion of patients in any case

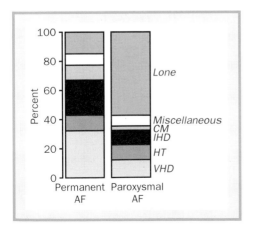

Figure 2
Associated cardiac diagnoses in patients with paroxysmal AF and permanent AF.
CM = cardiomyopathy; IHD = ischaemic heart disease; HT = hypertensive heart disease; VHD = valvular heart disease.
(Reproduced with permission from the *Lancet* (1993) 341: 1317–22)

series depends on the age and clinical characteristics of the study population. The frequency of lone AF is also dependent on the extent of screening investigations. In particular, echocardiography will detect asymptomatic valvular or myocardial dysfunction (although mild to moderate atrial dilatation may result from AF, and is allowed within the definition of lone AF). The diagnosis of lone AF should prompt consideration of newly recognized clinical types of AF, such as familial AF discussed above and 'focal AF' discussed in later chapters.

Asymptomatic AF is frequent (about one-third of all cases), and this fact is brought out in electrocardiographic surveys of populations, where many cases of undiagnosed and untreated AF are found. The initial detection of AF is often at health screening visits for hypertension. Preoperative examination often reveals previously undiagnosed AF. In addition many pacemaker patients have AV block and hence their transition to AF may be asymptomatic unless a dual chamber pacemaker responds to the onset of AF by pacing the ventricles rapidly. Finally, AF may first present with a devastating cerebrovascular accident. Some of the AF first noted after the occurrence of a stroke is transient, possibly because it is caused by the stroke (any devastating neurological event may cause cardiac arrhythmias) or is paroxysmal in nature.

Key references

1. Kannel WB, Abbott RD, Savage DD, McNamara PM. Epidemiologic features of atrial fibrillation. The Framingham study. *N Engl J Med* (1982) **306:** 1018–22.

2. Krahn AD, Manfreda J, Tate RB et al. The natural history of atrial fibrillation: incidence, risk factors, and prognosis in the Manitoba follow-up study. *Am J Med* (1995) **98:** 476–84.

3. Camm AJ, Obel OA. Epidemiology and mechanism of atrial fibrillation and atrial flutter. *Am J Cardiol* (1996) **78:** 3–11.

Morbidity and mortality of AF

3

Morbidity

Quality of life and symptoms

Apart from causing symptoms of palpitations, chest discomfort and breathlessness, the fast and irregular ventricular rates associated with AF can precipitate angina, cardiac failure, presyncope and occasionally syncope in susceptible patients. AF has a considerable impact on quality of life. This is best studied in the context of paroxysmal AF, when the patient can be interrogated in both sinus rhythm and in AF. Questionnaires may be repeated after interventions such as AV nodal ablation and implantation of a mode switching dual chamber pacemaker ('ablate and pace', a treatment strategy discussed in depth later). Interventional procedures for paroxysmal, persistent or permanent AF may dramatically reduce symptoms and improve quality of life.

The mechanism of symptoms in AF is poorly defined but relates to multiple haemodynamic and functional inefficiencies inherent in the arrhythmia. These are outlined in Figure 4, and the importance of each factor is dependent on the patient's characteristics. In those with diastolic

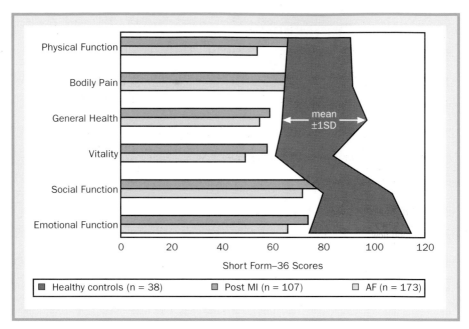

Figure 3
The impact of AF on quality of life. Six dimensions of the Short Form (SF) 36 are illustrated (unpublished data).

dysfunction the loss of atrial transport and reduced diastolic filling time are deleterious, while patients with coronary insufficiency suffer most from the reduction in diastolic coronary perfusion time and increased cardiac work from the tachycardia. Overall no clear-cut mechanisms are proven for individuals as all effects inherently coexist, but assessment of the probable dominant factor is important as it will determine therapeutic strategies. For example, pharmacological rate control reduces the ventricular rate, and the 'ablate and pace' strategy adds rhythm regularization, but neither therapy restores atrial transport.

Stroke

The predominant impact of AF on mortality is through its strong association with stroke. When associated with rheumatic heart disease, the risk of stroke in AF is seventeen times that of the general population. In recent years it has become

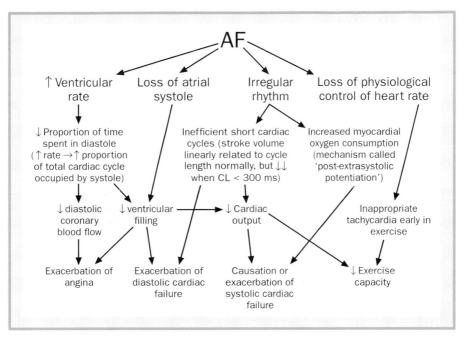

Figure 4
Haemodynamic and functional effects of AF.

apparent that even in the absence of underlying valvular heart disease, the risk is increased more than five-fold, and it has been estimated that 35% of patients with nonvalvular AF will eventually sustain a stroke if untreated. About 15% of ischaemic strokes arise as a consequence of AF, and more than half of cardiogenic embolic stroke is directly due to AF. Although many patients with AF have other risk factors for stroke such as aortic or carotid atherosclerosis, more than 70% of stroke in AF is due to embolism of thrombus from the left atrium. Approximately

90% of such left atrial thrombi arise within the left atrial appendage.

Thromboembolism in AF can also occur to other parts of the circulation including those supplied by the peripheral, renal and splenic vessels. There are clinical (Figure 5) and echocardiographic (Figure 6) predictors of those patients with AF who are particularly at risk of suffering a cerebrovascular accident. The latter include left atrial enlargement, left ventricular dysfunction, and the presence of

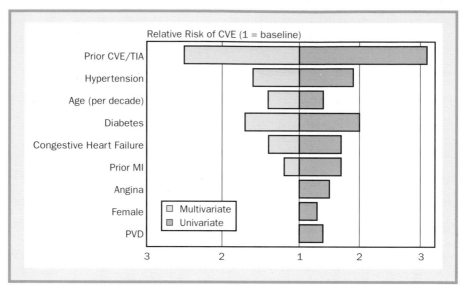

Figure 5
Univariate and multivariate predictors of stroke from a meta-analysis of five randomized trials.
(Arch Intern Med (1994) 154: 1449–57) CVE = cerbrovascular event; TIA = transient ischaemic attack;
MI = myocardial infarction; PVD = peripheral vascular disease.

left atrial thrombus or 'spontaneous echo contrast' on transoesophageal echocardiography. Mitral regurgitation somewhat reduces the risk of stroke, presumably because blood stasis is reduced by the high pressure backwash of blood into the left atrium.

Tachycardiomyopathy

The persistently high ventricular rates found with some AF are associated in an unknown proportion of cases with the development of a form of ventricular dilatation and dysfunction known as 'tachycardiomyopathy' (Figure 7). The recognition of this syndrome is important since many cases are fully or partially reversible with either cure of AF or improved ventricular rate control. The precise mechanism of developing this complication is poorly defined as it is only diagnosed retrospectively, when ventricular dilatation has occurred. However, it is clear that tachycardia is the major component and a mean

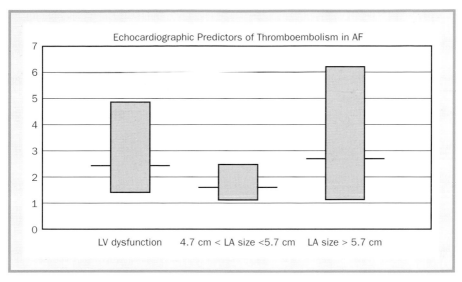

Figure 6
Echocardiographic predictors of stroke in the SPAF trial.
(Ann Int Med (1992) 116: 6–12) LV = left ventricle; LA = left atrium.

ventricular rate above 120 bpm, and probably higher is required. Improvement in left ventricular function following cardioversion or 'ablate and pace' treatment (see Chapter 9) suggests lower rates may also be deleterious. Tachycardiomyopathy is recognized in other tachycardias like incessant VT and junctional tachycardias.

Atrial fibrillation causes changes in the atria themselves. Progressive atrial dilatation occurs (Figure 8), probably due to an atrial tachycardiomyopathy which has cellular

mechanisms discussed in the next chapter, but also because of a rise in left atrial pressure which accompanies the onset of AF.

Mortality

The dominant mechanism of mortality in AF is thromboembolism to the brain causing stroke and, more rarely, fatal emboli to other sites (for example mesenteric emboli). AF related death from congestive cardiac failure may be due to exacerbation of existing pump failure or occasionally from

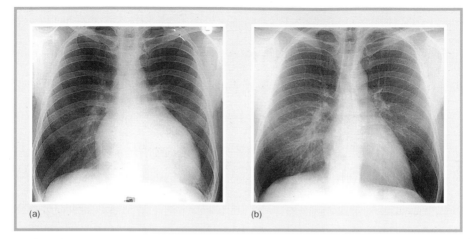

Figure 7
Chest X-rays from a patient who presented with AF and congestive cardiac failure. CXR (a) was taken at presentation, and (b) 2 months after sinus rhythm had been restored. Cardiac size was initially greatly increased, but reverted to normal with the resolution of the AF induced, tachycardia related cardiomyopathy ('AF tachycardiomyopathy').

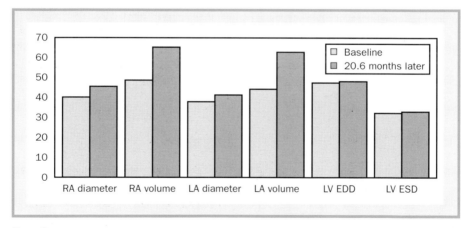

Figure 8
The effect of AF on atrial and ventricular size in 15 patients. Measurements were made 20.6 months apart. Atrial volumes are in cm³ and LV cavity dimensions in mm.
(Circulation (1990) 82: 792–7) RA = right atrium; LA = left atrium; LV = left ventricle; EDD = end diastolic diameter; ESD = end systolic diameter.

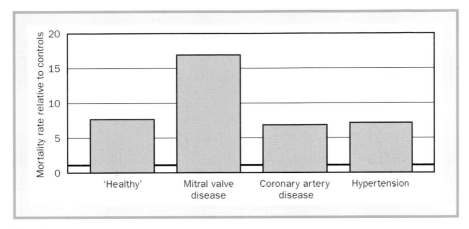

Figure 9
Mortality in an insured population: 3099 people accepted for life assurance. Figure shows mortality rates, relative to subjects without AF, for those without documented co-existent disease ('healthy' or lone AF), as well as those with known cardiovascular disease.
(JAMA (1981) 245: 1540–4)

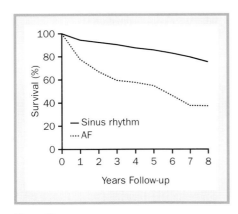

Figure 10
Survival during follow-up of patients with angiographically proven coronary artery disease according to cardiac rhythm.
(Am J Cardiol (1988) 61: 714–17)

tachycardiomyopathy solely due to AF. Sudden cardiac death can occur because the rapid irregular rhythm provokes ventricular arrythmias related to co-existent structural heart disease or antiarrhythmic drug therapy. Fatal drug related proarrhythmia may also occur during sinus rhythm.

AF is associated with a higher than expected death rate in those with coronary artery disease, hypertension, mitral valve disease and even apparently otherwise healthy persons (Figure 9). The occurrence of AF is predictive of a worse outcome in those with chronic stable angina (Figure 10) and following myocardial infarction (Figure 11). Patients with congestive cardiac

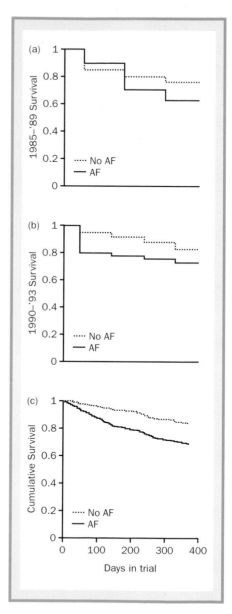

Figure 11
1-year mortality after myocardial infarction according to cardiac rhythm.
(Br Heart J *(1978) 40: 303–7)*

failure who suffer from AF are also thought to have a worse outcome (Figure 12). The increased mortality rate for these diverse patient groups is due in part to patients with AF having more severe disease (or subclinical diseases in the case of 'healthy subjects'), but after careful adjustment for risk factors, all-cause mortality is still higher than sinus rhythm controls.

Figure 12
Mortality amongst patients with severe heart failure according to cardiac rhythm; (a) and (b) are taken from two cohorts based upon treatment years. From 1985 to 1989 there was a markedly worse survival amongst those with AF, but this was much less striking (and no longer statistically significant) by 1990 to 1993.
The authors (Stevenson et al. JACC (1996) 28: 1458–63) *attribute this to wider use of ACE inhibitors and amiodarone, and reduced use of other antiarrhythmics. Other recent data (c), however, suggests AF is still an important predictor of mortality in CHF.* (Konety et al. Circ (1988) 98: I–703)

Conclusion

AF is associated with significant morbidity and mortality which can easily be overlooked since, as with cerebral thromboembolism, complications often occur remote from the onset of the arrhythmia, and may not easily be attributed to it. Furthermore, AF is associated with other diseases such as heart failure, which have an important independent impact on survival. The importance of AF is clearly recognizable but most of the data are retrospective and collected primarily for other purposes. Prospective data are needed on aspects ranging from mortality to long-term efficacy of treatment strategies.

Key references

1. Brignole M, Gianfranchi L, Menozzi C et al. Assessment of atrioventricular junction ablation and DDDR mode-switching pacemaker versus pharmacological treatment in patients with severely symptomatic paroxysmal atrial fibrillation: a randomized controlled study. *Circulation* (1997) **96:** 2617–24.

2. Daoud EG, Weiss R, Bahu M et al. Effect of an irregular ventricular rhythm on cardiac output. *Am J Cardiol* (1996) **78:** 1433–6.

3. Kerr C, Boone J, Connolly S et al. Follow-up of atrial fibrillation: the initial experience of the Canadian Registry of Atrial Fibrillation. *Eur Heart J* (1996) **17** (Supplement C): 48–51.

4. Benjamin EJ, Wolf PA, D'Agostino RB et al. Impact of atrial fibrillation on risk of death: the Framingham Heart study. *Circulation* (1998) **98:** 946 –52.

Atrial structure and function

4

Atrial fibrillation is associated with several anatomical, morphological and pathological abnormalities in the atria. As with many features of this disease, these may be caused by or be the result of the disorder. Often the precise interrelationship, particularly in individuals, is not fully delineated.

The effect of age on atrial myocardium

The prevalence of AF rises steeply with increasing age, and aging itself is associated with changes in the atrial histology. Elastic tissue and collagen replaces a proportion of atrial muscle. This increase in electrically inert tissue also occurs in the region of the sinus node, is accompanied by loss of sinus node pacemaker (P) cells, and increases the propensity to develop sick sinus syndrome, which is commonly associated with AF. Diffuse deposits of a birefringent tissue within the atrial myocardium and sinus node area also occur with increased aging. This amyloid-like tissue is probably denatured atrial naturetic peptide. These changes cause slowing and fragmentation of sinus impulses as they conduct through the atria and predispose individuals to the development of AF.

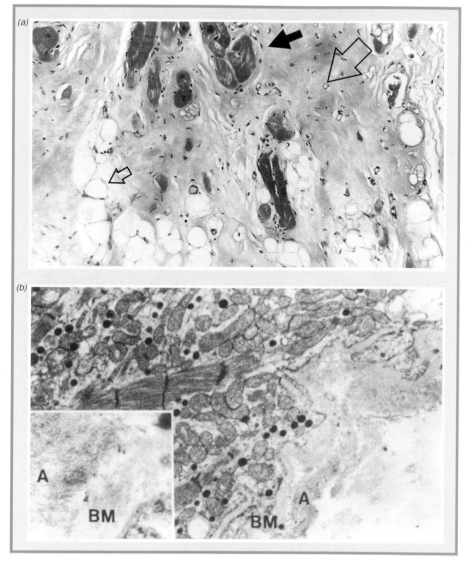

Figure 13
*Atrial histology in AF. (a) Sparse atrial myocytes (dark arrow), adipocytes (small open arrows) and fibrous
tissue (large open arrows). In normal subjects, the latter two are largely absent. (b) Atrial amyloid.
A = amyloid tissue; B = basement membrane. (Reproduced with permission from* Br Heart J *(1986)
56:17–20)*

Specific atrial disease processes

AF generally represents an end-stage response to disease and degenerative processes. Any disease inducing atrial dilatation (through pressure or volume overload), atrial scarring or atrial ischaemia can predispose to AF. However, AF may be the result of specific inflammatory or infiltrative disorders, which are in some cases confined to the heart, or even to the atria alone. Some data suggest that an inflammatory myopathy is present in two-thirds of cases of 'lone' AF, with active myocarditis in a quarter of cases. Antimyosin antibodies have also been detected in some patients with paroxysmal AF. It is currently unclear if these autoantibodies against the

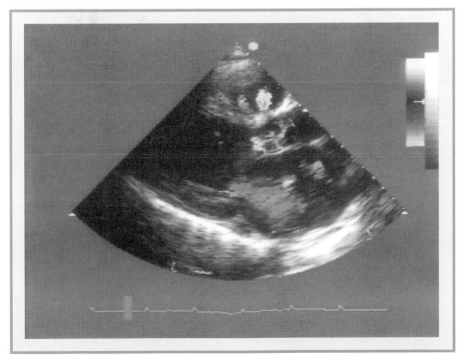

Figure 14
Echo showing an enlarged left atrium and a jet of mitral regurgitation. Interestingly, mitral regurgitation appears to provide partial protection against left atrial thrombus formation and hence against stroke. However, the effect is not marked enough to remove the need for warfarin.
(The colouring of this image has been modified for technical reasons.)

cardiac muscle protein play a role in the causation of AF or are a result of fibrillation-induced atrial muscle damage.

More established diseases leading to AF include rheumatic carditis, neoplastic conditions such as primary atrial myxoma and secondary metastases from distant sites, sarcoidosis, and primary cardiac amyloidosis. Arteritis as occurs in systemic lupus erythematosis (SLE) can cause focal necrosis and subsequent fibrosis of atrial tissue which can result in AF. Dilated and hypertrophic cardiomyopathy may induce AF, presumably because of changes secondary to impaired systolic or diastolic left ventricular function, usually occurring relatively late in the disease. However, when AF occurs as an early manifestation of the disease process a specific atrial myopathic process is suspected.

Changes resulting from AF

AF itself induces morphological and pathological changes in the atria. The onset of AF is associated with left atrial pressure rise, and in the long term, left atrial dilatation occurs (Figure 8). At the histological level mitochondrial swelling, cell death and fibrosis are seen, and may be mediated by intracellular calcium overload. Such changes may result in a self-perpetuating cycle by promoting further AF.

Key references

1. Davies MJ, Pomerance A. Pathology of atrial fibrillation in man. *Br Heart J* (1972) **34:** 520–5.

2. Frustaci A, Chimenti C, Bellocci F et al. Histological substrate of atrial biopsies in patients with lone atrial fibrillation. *Circulation* (1997) **96:** 1180–4.

3. Ausma J, Wijffels M, Thone F et al. Structural changes of atrial myocardium due to sustained atrial fibrillation in the goat. *Circulation* (1997) **96:** 3157–63.

4. Manning WJ, Silverman DI. Atrial anatomy and function postcardioversion: insights from transthoracic and transesophageal echocardiography. *Prog Cardiovasc Dis* (1996) **39:** 33–46.

Electrophysiology

5

Three basic mechanisms are responsible for the genesis of cardiac arrhythmias: (1) re-entry; (2) enhanced automaticity; and (3) triggered activity. Originally it was thought that AF was due to multifocal atrial activity but it is now accepted that AF is usually perpetualized by a re-entrant arrhythmia. Unlike most re-entrant arrhythmias however, which involve a

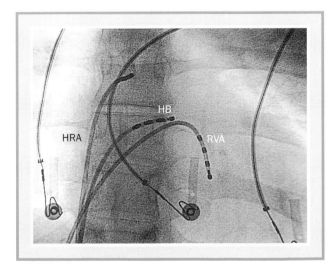

Figure 15
A three-wire electrophysiological study in an AF patient. Wires are positioned at the right ventricular apex (RVA), His bundle (HB) and high right atrium (HRA). Depending on the precise goal of the study, more wires may be employed: in the coronary sinus, positioned transseptally or retrogradely in the left atrium, or a multielectrode basket catheter may be used.

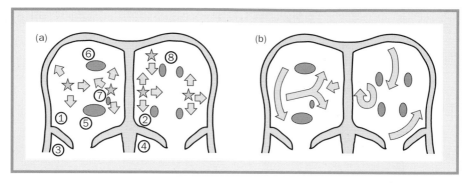

Figure 16
(a) AF was once thought to be due entirely to multifocal discharge, but it is now recognized to be due to multiple wavelet re-entry (b). ① is the right atrium and ② is the left. ③ and ④ are right and left ventricles. Also shown are the inferior ⑤ and superior ⑥ venae cavae, the coronary sinus ⑦ and the pulmonary veins ⑧.

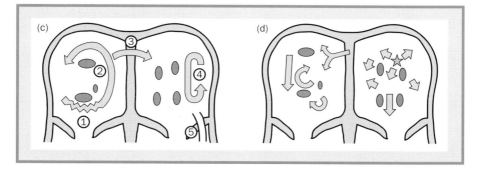

Over time (c), the importance of zones of slow conduction ①, stable rotors ②, specialized conduction tracts ③, tissue anisotropy ④ and concomitant arrhythmias such as AVRT ⑤ have become appreciated. Recently (d), focal atrial tachycardia (★) and fibrillatory conduction to the rest of the atria has been documented as the cause of AF in some patients.

single fixed re-entrant circuit, AF results from multiple interlacing or randomly meandering re-entrant 'wavelets'.

The more wavelets that are present within the atria, the less the likelihood of their simultaneous extinction and, therefore, the

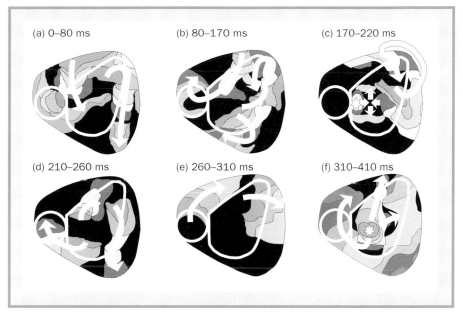

Figure 17
An isochronal map of AF. In each figure, an increasing depth of colour indicates progressively later activation within 50 ms time windows. Black areas are not activated during the period under study. The white arrows are a graphic representation of the progression of wavefronts of depolarization. As can be appreciated, there is random wavelet re-entry. In the final frame (f), there is the appearance of a new area of depolarization which may represent a spontaneous local discharge or, more likely, an endocardial breakthrough of a wavelet that had been travelling on the epicardium.
(Adapted from Cardiac Electrophysiology and Arrhythmias. *Grune & Stratton: London, 1984 with permission)*

less likely that AF will terminate. In order to accommodate multiple wavelets the atria must be large (explaining the association of AF with atrial dilatation) or the wavelets short. The wavelength is the theoretical minimum distance that can be travelled by the wave of depolarization while still allowing it to 're-enter'.

It is calculated by multiplying the conduction velocity by the refractory period (Figure 18).

Over time, the importance of other electrophysiological phenomena have become appreciated. AF is associated with increased dispersion of refractory periods within the

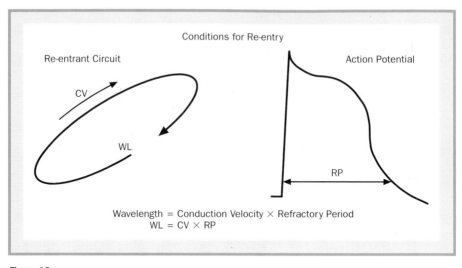

Figure 18
Wavelength is the product of conduction velocity and refractory period.

atria, fragmented atrial activity (disorganized atrial activity recorded in atrial electrograms), and repetitive atrial firing in response to a single premature stimulus (reflecting an increased tendency to triggered activity). Anisotropic conduction, which is faster and more reliable conduction along the long axis of cardiac muscle fibres than perpendicular to their orientation, is important in the creation of functional block (around which wavelets can rotate) and slow conduction. Certain functional circuits and 'specialized' conduction tracts (in practice, large muscle bundles; there is no conduction system corresponding to the His–Purkinje system of the ventricles) have proven to be important. These include Bachmann's bundle, connecting the left and right atria, and the crista terminalis, which runs vertically in the posterior right atrium just anterior to the venae cavae. At the histological level, myocardial discontinuities produced by fibrosis or by dilatation, also cause separation of muscle fascicles, enhancing anisotropy and resulting in slow disorganized and fragmented conduction.

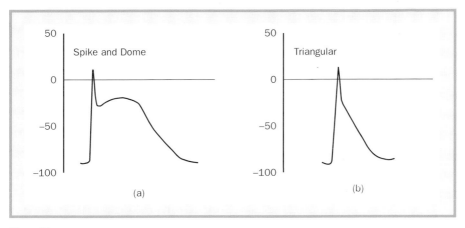

Figure 19
A normal atrial action potential (a) and following 2 weeks of AF (b). Although both types of action potential occur normally, the triangular form is predominant in AF.

Recent findings indicate that AF results in a 'remodelling' of the electrophysiological properties of the atrium. In particular, the refractory period becomes progressively shorter such that wavelets become smaller and make room for more wavelets. The atrial fibrillation becomes more stable and less likely to convert to sinus rhythm. The fact that the atrial remodelling process leads to perpetuation of the arrhythmia has led to the concept that 'atrial fibrillation *begets* atrial fibrillation'. This remodelling is reflected in the atrial action potential which tends to become triangular and foreshortened (Figure 19).

AF occurs in association with other arrhythmias. The incidence of AF in patients with AV re-entrant tachycardia (AVRT, the WPW syndrome) and AV nodal re-entrant tachycardia (AVNRT) is much higher than expected by chance. Atrial flutter often co-exists with AF, with some patients switching between the two arrhythmias during paroxysmal episodes. At electrophysiological study, there may be fibrillation of the left atrium with organized regular activity on the right, akin to that seen during flutter. The nature of the interaction between sick sinus syndrome and AF is slightly different. In many, but not all, cases of sick sinus syndrome there is a diffuse or multifocal atrial disease process and AF occurs in a substantial proportion of cases. It can provide the tachycardia element of the so-called

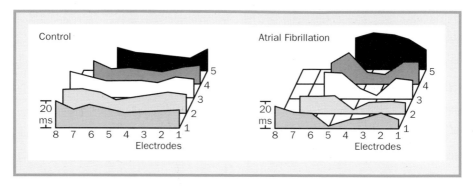

Figure 20
A comparison of the dispersion of atrial refractoriness in normal subjects and those who suffer from AF. Recordings were made from up to eight electrodes from catheters in five different places in the atria. The height of the line represents the local refractory period. AF sufferers have much more variability with some areas having a very short refractory period. (J Am Coll Cardiol (1992) 19(7): 1531–5)

tachycardia–bradycardia syndrome, which is a clinical subtype of sick sinus syndrome.

Recently, some patients who suffer from AF clinically have been found to have a single atrial focus that causes the condition. This fires so rapidly that conduction to the rest of the atrium breaks down and may give rise to re-entrant, self-sustaining waves akin to AF. Currently it seems that this is what accounts for a minor proportion of AF, but the true incidence is unknown and may be much higher. This mechanism is very important because an arrhythmogenic focus can be located and ablated thus leading to a clinical cure for the arrhythmia.

Conclusion: triggers and maintenance

Concepts regarding the electrophysiology of AF are changing, particularly since the description of 'focal AF'. The elucidation of this mechanism has led to a distinction between those processes which initiate (and re-initiate), and those that perpetuate or sustain AF. Distinct mechanisms that induce termination of AF have not yet been defined. Once AF occurs, it is usually maintained by multiple wavelet re-entry. Improved understanding has led to refinement of the original hypothesis. Alterations to atrial electrophysiology by the AF itself and other disease processes may promote continuation of the arrhythmia. Triggering of the arrhythmia may be by other tachycardias, repeated atrial ectopics, alterations in autonomic tone or external triggers such as myocardial infarction or pneumonia. The concept has clinical relevance: patients with paroxysmal AF have frequent triggers to AF but maintain it poorly, while those with persistent AF maintain the arrhythmia well, but only suffer infrequent triggering (see Chapter 6 for detailed discussion of classification).

Summary of electrophysiological changes associated with atrial fibrillation:

(1)   Rapid repolarisation of atrial tissue (short refractory period).

(2)   Areas of slow conduction (reduced conduction velocity).

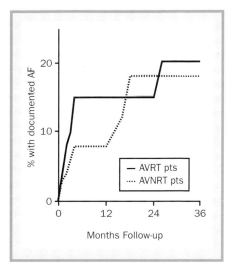

Figure 21
The cumulative incidence of documented AF in 167 patients with regular narrow complex tachycardia. Prior to the study, AF had been found in only 12 of the patients.
(Hamer et al. J Am Coll Cardiol (1995) 25: 984–8)

Features Favouring Diagnostic EP Study
• Documented regular tachycardia
• Pre-excitation on the resting ECG
• Control of AF difficult (resistance to multiple antiarrhythmics)
• Young patients
• Lone AF patients
• Evidence of focal AF (stereotypical onset, frequent PACs and runs of atrial tachycardia)

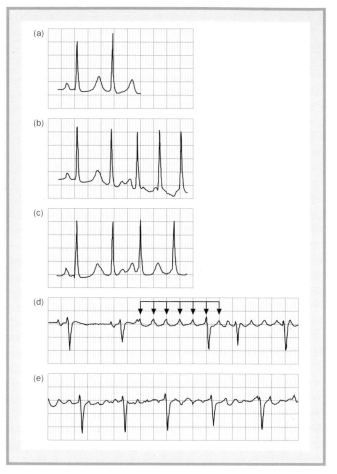

Figure 22
Holter example of probable focal AF. In patient 1, there were frequent atrial ectopics (a) seen during the Holter. Two episodes of AF occurred, both preceded by the same ectopic (b and c), and the following atrial activity and RR coupling interval were identical for both episodes. In (d) and (e), from another patient, the RR interval pattern at AF onset is not reproducible, but there is regular atrial activation at the start of AF episodes. (d) shows AF onset with an atrial tachycardia, degenerating into AF in (e).

(3) Short wavelength (product of above two factors).

(4) Increased dispersion of refractory periods, anisotropy and delayed, fractionated and abnormal conduction (particularly important in areas which form barriers to conduction such as the crista terminalis, or block of conduction pathways such as Bachman's Bundle).

(5) Repetitive atrial firing (spontaneously or in response to a premature stimulus).

(6) Other re-entrant or focal tachycardias such as AVRT, AVNRT, atrial flutter and atrial tachycardia.

(7) Sinus node dysfunction.

(8) Associated AV nodal and His Purkinje conduction disease.

Key references

1. Moe GK, Abildskov JA. Atrial fibrillation as a self-sustaining arrhythmia independent of focal discharge. *Am Heart J* (1959) **58:** 59–70.

2. Allessie MA, Konings K, Kirchhof CJ, Wijffels M. Electrophysiologic mechanisms of perpetuation of atrial fibrillation. *Am J Cardiol* (1996) **77:** 10A–23A.

3. Konings K, Kirchhof CJ, Smeets JRLM et al. High-density mapping of electrically induced atrial fibrillation in humans. *Circulation* (1994) **89:** 1665–80.

4. Wijffels M, Kirchhof CJ, Dorland R, Allessie MA. Atrial fibrillation begets atrial fibrillation: a study in awake chronically instrumented goats. *Circulation* (1995) **92:** 1954–68.

5. Jais P, Haissaguerre M, Shah DC et al. A focal source of atrial fibrillation treated by discrete radiofrequency ablation. *Circulation* (1997) **95:** 572–6.

6. Haissaguerre M, Jais P, Shah DC et al. Spontaneous initiation of atrial fibrillation by ectopic beats originating in the pulmonary veins. *N Engl J Med* (1998) **339:** 959–66.

Classification

6

Several overlapping systems are used to classify AF but such schemes are clinically useful only when the categories require different management. AF may be classified according to its aetiology and underlying disease, its electrophysiological features or its temporal pattern.

When rheumatic heart disease accounted for most cases of AF in younger people, it was usual to divide it into rheumatic and nonrheumatic varieties. This nomenclature is less useful now, but AF is still divided into valvular and nonvalvular cases. Other aetiologies are used to categorize AF: ischaemic, alcoholic and thyrotoxic are useful because they focus attention on the need to deal with the underlying disease rather than the AF alone. Postoperative AF is also a useful separate category; it follows cardiac or thoracic surgery, carries a particularly low risk of thromboembolism and has a lesser tendency to recur after cardioversion. Most patients who have self-terminating paroxysms of AF do not have associated structural heart disease and the autonomic nervous system may have an important role in precipitating the condition in such cases. A clinical subgroup of patients with paroxysmal AF exists in which attacks occur at times of parasympathetic

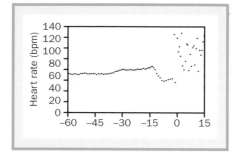

Figure 23
A typical tachogram from a patient with vagotonic AF. The AF onset follows a slowing of the sinus rate and has a slow mean ventricular rate.

dominance. So-called vagotonic AF typically affects younger patients, occurs in postprandial or evening or nocturnal paroxysms, tends not to progress to established forms of AF, and usually occurs with a slow ventricular rate. 'Adrenergic AF' is also described, where attacks occur during or after exercise and the AF often associated with mild to moderate structural heart disease. Perhaps as much as one quarter of paroxysmal AF is vagotonic or mostly vagotonic, and one fifth is adrenergic or predominantly adrenergic. Many patients present mixed or indeterminate patterns.

Table 5
The features of vagotonic and adrenergenic AF

Vagatonic AF	Adrenergic AF
Younger (30 to 50 yr)	Older (50+ yr)
Male>Female	No gender bias
'Normal heart'	Structural heart disease
Post-prandial episodes	Episodes during or after exercise
Evening or nocturnal attacks	Early morning attacks
Slow ventricular rates in AF	Fast rates
Antecedent bradycardia	Prior tachycardia
Therapy	
Disopyramide	Propafenone
Class 1 antiarrhythmic agents	Sotalol
Atrial pacing	Beta blockers
(Aggravated by digoxin)	

The distinction 'coarse' from 'fine' AF, based on the amplitude of the fibrillation waves on the surface ECG, predicts response to treatment but its discriminatory power is poor. Coarse AF (i.e. high amplitude fibrillation waves, $\geqslant 2$ mm in V_1) has the worse outcome. Systems of classification based on intracardiac or surface electrograms exist, but are only useful in a research setting.

Until the development of effective cardioversion AF could follow only one of two temporal patterns: self-terminating paroxysms alternating with sinus rhythm, or permanent AF. Cardioversion creates a third pattern, in which episodes are terminated by DC shock (or drug therapy) but tend to not terminate spontaneously — so-called persistent AF (Figure 24).

Once chronic, AF is classified as paroxysmal, persistent or permanent, but when it first arises, it is unclear whether it is transient, recurrent or chronic. In this situation the term 'first onset' AF is useful. Many patients will suffer a solitary episode of AF in the context of an acute illness such as myocardial infarction or an alcohol binge but for them it may not be a long-term problem.

The classification of different forms of chronic AF is important. Assignment to permanent rather than persistent AF may be determined by prior history. For example multiple failed

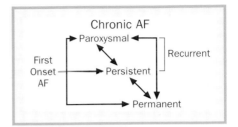

Figure 24
The progression from first onset to chronic AF, and the possible movement between the 3 Ps: paroxysmal (repeated attacks of self-terminating attacks of AF); persistent (AF that does not revert spontaneously but will do so with medical intervention) and permanent (AF that either will not cardiovert, or it is not appropriate to try to revert to sinus rhythm).

cardioversions despite drug prophylaxis. However the physician also has a role in the less clear-cut cases to determine whether attempts at restoring sinus rhythm are in the patient's interests: in many patients 'permanent' AF is allowed without any attempt to cardiovert. It should be an active decision not to pursue restoration of sinus rhythm, and chosen only when there is no likelihood of clinical gain to the patient. These management decisions and others are influenced by whether the patient has lone AF or if there is associated cardiac or noncardiac disease. With time the importance of permanent AF as a clinical subtype will dwindle as treatments improve. AF may move between classes over time (Figure 25) and both paroxysmal and persistent AF alternate

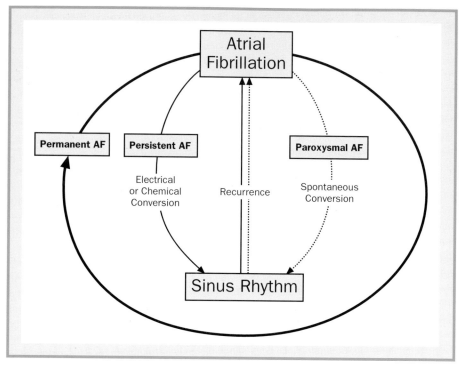

Figure 25
A system of classification based on the time course of AF.

with normal sinus rhythm. About 30% of paroxysmal AF becomes established (persistent or permanent) in 1 year, but some cases do not progress over many years. Even in those who remain paroxysmal, the intensity of their arrhythmia waxes and wanes over time.

- First onset AF: evaluate cause and restore sinus rhythm if necessary.

- Paroxysmal AF: prevent episodes and/or minimize their symptomatic impact.

- Persistent AF: restore sinus rhythm and prevent recurrences of AF.

- Permanent AF: control the ventricular rate and restore a regular rhythm to improve symptoms and prognosis.

Table 6
Summary of the pros and cons of attempting to maintain sinus rhythm versus accepting permanent AF. The balance will shift further in favour of sinus rhythm as treatments improve (e.g. curative RF ablation, implantable atrioverters, and safe and effective drug therapy).

	Sinus Rhythm with Recurrent Persistent AF	Permanent AF
Anticoagulation	Only during AF and post-cardioversion	Lifelong
Atrial transport and chronotropic response	Normal (but atrial mechanical dysfunction and sinus disease not infrequent)	Lost (near-normalization of chronotropic response possible by drugs or rate responsive pacemaker)
Exercise tolerance	Normal	Reduced by 20 to 30% on average
AF symptoms	Only when AF recurs	Constant
Interventions and hospitalizations	Each time AF recurs	Infrequent
Antiarrhythmic therapy	Needed for most after first AF recurrence (proarrhythmic risks)	Not indicated
Efficacy of strategy	Permanent AF occurs in a significant proportion over 2–5 years but therapies are improving	Rate control is possible by drugs or AV nodal ablation. Anticoagulants are contraindicated in some.

As discussed later, the type of AF substantially affects the risk of thromboembolism.

Key reference

Gallagher MG, Camm AJ. Classification of atrial fibrillation. *Pacing Clin Electrophysiol* (1997) **20:** 1603–5.

Evaluation

7

Evaluation of a patient with AF must first consider whether there is an important underlying disease. The onset of AF may be due to a life threatening condition such as dilated cardiomyopathy or metastatic carcinoma, or to other important diseases such as thyrotoxicosis. Next the current symptomatic and clinical impact of the AF may be assessed, and the risk of future complications estimated (Table 8). Physician evaluation provides much of the information and clinical factors largely determine whether:

(a) The patient should be cardioverted immediately or later;

(b) The ventricular rate should be reduced acutely or over the long term;

(c) Anticoagulation is needed acutely or in the long term.

Any patient who is to have active management of their AF requires fuller evaluation through appropriate investigation.

Table 7
Investigations and their possible findings in AF.

Investigation	Purpose
Echocardiogram	Define LA size and LV function. Exclude valvular disease
FBC	Exclude anaemia contributing to dyspnoea
U+E's	Check potassium and renal function
LFT	Evidence of ethanol intake
TFT	Hyperthyroidism found in 1%, but very important
12 lead ECG	Resting ventricular rate, old MI's and accessory pathways
Holter recording	Asymptomatic arrhythmias, rate control
Exercise test	Co-existent ischaemia, rate control, exercise induced arrhythmias
Event recorder	Document arrhythmias
CXR	Co-existent lung pathology, baseline CTR
EP study	Identify treatable arrhythmias
Cardiac catheter	Evaluate co-existent coronary and valve disease

FBC = full blood count; U+E's = urea and electrolytes; LFT = liver function tests; TFT = thyroid function tests; CXR = chest X-ray; EP = electrophysiology; LA = left atrium; LV = left ventricle; MI = myocardial infarction; CTR = cardiothoracic ratio.

Clinical assessment

The history and clinical examination dictate the nature and extent of further investigation. The causes and complications of AF as well as the evaluation of optimal treatment are all important. Therefore the possible range of investigations is very extensive.

Ongoing ethanol abuse reduces the probability of successful long-term AF control, and careful documentation of ethanol intake is important. It is worthwhile checking the γ G T-level to guide initial advice and for subsequent reference. While a high intake of ethanol is undoubtedly harmful, the effect of a moderate consumption is unclear. Patients

Table 8
Tests for the evaluation of a patient with AF. Other investigations such as chest X-ray and coronary angiography may also
be indicated.

Aims of evaluation	History and examination	Blood tests	Echo-cardiogram	Ambulatory ECG (Holter recording)	Exercise Tolerance Test
Rule out underlying disease requiring treatment	+ +	+ +	+ +		+
Decide whether to convert to sinus rhythm	+ +		+		
Decide whether to give long-term anticoagulant therapy	+ +		+		
Fully evaluate the AF and its symptoms, including determining ventricular rate control	+ +			I I	+ +

+ + Very important, almost always involved in decision; + usually used, sometimes to answer a specific question.

should be advised to reduce their intake to within the recommended range and to avoid 'binge drinking'. If AF control proves difficult, complete abstinence, for a period of at least several months, should be strongly recommended. However, if this makes no difference to the incidence of the AF this instruction should be relaxed.

Many cases of AF are discovered incidentally at, for example, blood pressure screening visits and are thought to be asymptomatic. While some patients may not have symptoms, more often the symptoms are not perceived. Physicians tend to focus on palpitations as the most important feature of AF but patients are often more aware of exertional dyspnoea, poor exercise tolerance and lethargy. Therefore, the true impact of the disease may be missed. Even with patients who claim to be asymptomatic, a substantial improvement in exercise tolerance and general well-being is

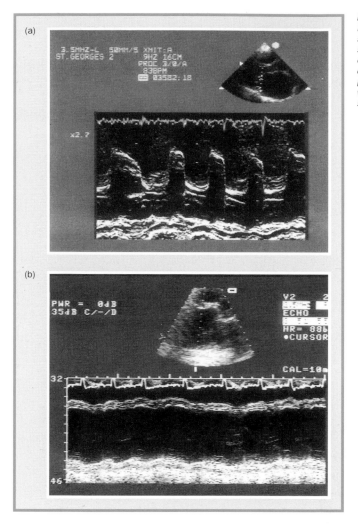

Figure 26
Echocardiograms
showing (a) mitral
stenosis and (b) M-mode
of moderate LV
dysfunction in AF
patients. Both findings
were not clinically
suspected.

usually reported following successful cardioversion. Asymptomatic patients are probably as much at risk of thromboembolism as others. Because they are unaware of their cardiac rhythm, they may develop a significant tachycardia and be at risk of tachycardia-induced cardiomyopathy.

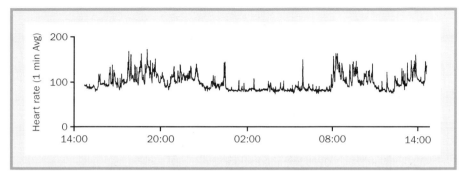

Figure 27
Holter tachogram showing poor ventricular rate control despite a combination of digoxin and verapamil. This patient eventually went on to have an AV nodal ablation with implantation of a rate responsive pacemaker.

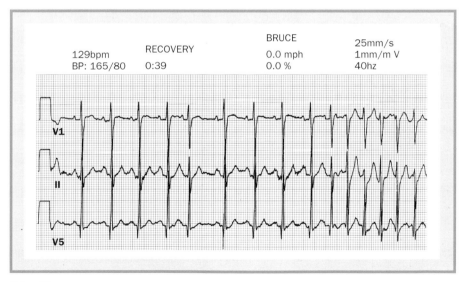

Figure 28
Short runs of AF during the recovery stage of an exercise test in a patient with negative Holter studies and other investigations.

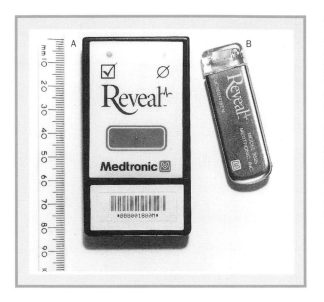

Figure 29
The Medtronic 'Reveal' implantable loop recorder is inserted using a minor surgical procedure. It is currently used for diagnosing the cause of syncope, but can potentially be used for any infrequent paroxysmal rhythm disturbance or for other rhythm monitoring purposes. A current multicentre study is evaluating the device in AF patients. Later generations of this device are likely to be specially designed for the monitoring of AF: occurrence of paroxysms, daily heart rate profiles, etc. The patient triggers the implanted device (B) with an external activator (A).

In patients who suffer from self-terminating paroxysms of AF, palpitations are usually the dominant symptom. Some are unaware of their cardiac rhythm and therefore present with episodic presyncope, effort dyspnoea or chest pain. Clinical symptoms cannot be relied upon to differentiate paroxysmal from continuous AF as some patients complain of episodic palpitations despite AF being constantly present (intermittently symptomatic AF). This is an important clinical subgroup that may confuse the physician who might only observe an arrythmia when symptoms arise and assume that sinus rhythm is present when the AF is clinically silent.

Investigations

Proper evaluation of the 12-lead ECG is vital. First the diagnosis must be confirmed, as confusion may arise from other causes of an irregular pulse, particularly in those with atrial flutter and complete heart block. In AF, the baseline shows low amplitude irregular fibrillation waves with an irregularly irregular ventricular rhythm. Conversely, a regular pulse may be found in patients with AF and baseline activity may be mimicked by myopotential noise or poor skin preparation, or masked by a low amplitude signal (for example obesity) or an over-filtered ECG signal. Coarse fibrillation waves may be

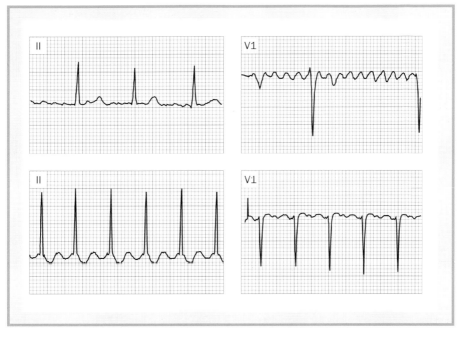

Figure 30
The top traces of atrial fibrillation illustrate the relatively high amplitude of 'F' waves in V1 (compared to lead II). Conversely, the lower traces show that atrial flutter signals ('F' waves) are bigger in II than in lead V1.

mistaken for atrial flutter, but the two can be differentiated by the truly irregular response in AF (flutter typically exhibits 2:1 block, occasionally 3:1 or 4:1, and rarely variable block but is not usually completely irregular) and the fact that flutter is best seen in inferior leads (II, III and aVF) while AF signals typically have the highest amplitude in V1 (Figure 30). AF may co-exist with complete heart block where AF is visible as the baseline, but the ventricular rhthym is very slow and

regular. Finally, other abnormalities such as Q waves, left ventricular hypertrophy, axis deviation and low amplitude ventricular complexes may give clues to co-existent disease.

Essential blood tests include a full blood count, serum electrolytes and thyroid function, and often a serum cholesterol is warranted. Thyrotoxicosis is a rare cause of AF, accounting for only 1–2% of new cases of

AF, but important because cardioversion and long-term maintenance of sinus rhythm is unlikely as long as the underlying condition persists. In some there are no or only subtle signs of an overactive thyroid, so-called 'apathetic hyperthyroidism', and AF is the only clinical marker of the disease. Anaemia may contribute to dyspnoea found in AF patients, and the white cell count may give a clue to lung sepsis that precipitated AF or suggest another inflammatory mechanism. Measures of the acute phase response such as ESR and CRP may give further guidance where inflammatory or malignant processes are suspected. Serum liver enzyme levels, and in particular γ GT, may be helpful when alcohol is suspected as a cause of AF.

Echocardiography is essential if active management is contemplated. Valve lesions, severe enough to cause AF, are usually evident on clinical examination, but may not be discovered. Echocardiography can detect left atrial dilatation (a giant left atrium may sometimes cause dysphagia, but atrial dilatation is usually asymptomatic) and subclinical left ventricular dysfunction. Both of these significantly increase the risk of stroke and reduce the likelihood of successful cardioversion.

Holter recordings may detect regular tachycardias or other information pertinent to the management of paroxysmal AF such as the ventricular rate during episodes of AF. In permanent AF, a Holter is necessary if there is doubt over the adequacy of ventricular rate control or to assess the cardiac rhythm during symptoms which are only intermittently present. Treadmill testing can precipitate adrenergic forms of paroxysmal AF and is also useful for assessing exercise ventricular rate control in active patients with permanent AF. It can be used to detect co-existing myocardial ischaemia, but interpretation of the exercise ECG in AF is difficult, especially if the patient is taking digoxin. Deferment until after cardioversion is therefore preferable, but if the diagnosis is required immediately nuclear medicine techniques or angiography are valuable.

Key references

1. Van den Berg MP, Tuinenburg AE, Crijns HJ et al. Heart failure and atrial fibrillation: current concepts and controversies. *Heart* (1997) **77:** 309–13.

2. Ettinger PO, Wu CF, De La Cruz C et al. Arrhythmias and the holiday heart: alcohol associated cardiac rhythm disorders. *Am Heart J* (1978) **95:** 555–62.

3. Nakazawa HK, Handa S, Nakamura Y et al. High maintenance rate of sinus rhythm after cardioversion in post-thyrotoxic chronic atrial fibrillation. *Int J Cardiol* (1987) **16:** 47–55.

Management

8

Four aspects of the management of atrial fibrillation are important.

(1) Rate control for permanent AF (long-term) or for first onset or paroxysmal/persistent forms (short-term).

(2) Cardioversion (electrical or pharmacological) for persistent or first onset AF.

(3) Prophylactic therapy to prevent recurrences of persistent or paroxysmal AF.

(4) Anticoagulation or antiplatelet therapy to minimize the risk from thromboembolic disease.

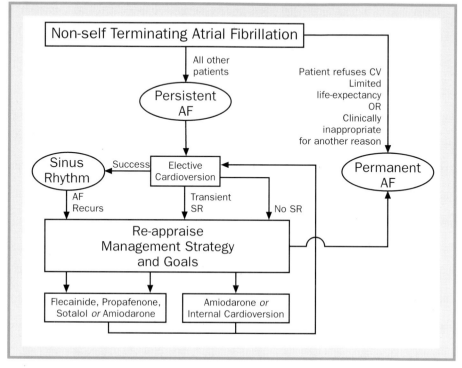

Figure 31
The management of AF which does not spontaneously terminate. An active decision is made as to whether to cardiovert. If cardioversion fails or if AF recurs, treatment goals are reappraised. If accepting permanent AF is rejected, additional therapy is offered (CV = cardioversion).

Because of a lingering but over optimistic concept that atrial fibrillation is essentially benign, therapy is often prescribed without sufficient evaluation of its need or its result. Physicians are too often prepared to accept that AF is permanent and do not try to restore sinus rhythm, cardioversion attempts are often half-hearted, the degree of rate control is never assessed, echocardiography is not performed to assess left ventricular function or thromboembolic risk, etc.

In any patient with AF, a potential cause of the arrhythmia must be sought and underlying disease must be identified and treated where possible, for example, hypertension and hyperthyroidism should be corrected and alcohol should be proscribed. The presence of underlying disease, while not necessarily causative or easily treatable, is also relevant for the assessment of thromboembolic risk. For example, a previous myocardial infarction, while not reversible by treatment, does add to the risk of thromboembolism and its presence must be considered when deciding whether to prescribe anticoagulants.

When evaluating the treatment of AF the physician is generally faced with a patient who is in sinus rhythm or in AF. When the patient is in sinus rhythm several important questions must be addressed.

- How many episodes of atrial fibrillation have been suffered by the patient?
- What is the usual duration of the episodes?
- How symptomatic was the patient during the attacks?
- Did the episodes terminate spontaneously or because of an intervention?
- Has any prophylactic therapy been tried, and with what result?
- Is there any change in the pattern of AF attacks (more frequent, longer lasting, more refractory, etc.)?

Primary Failure of External Cardioversion	Recurrence of AF after Successful Cardioversion
• Inadequate energy and poor technique	• Long duration of AF (more than 6 months)
• Obesity	• Dilated left atrium
• Hyperinflated chest (emphysema)	• Reduced LV function
• Long duration of AF (more than 6 months)	• Other structural heart disease (LV hypertrophy or valvular disease)
• Dilated left atrium	• Uncorrected hyperthyroidism and excess ethanol
	• Old age

Although broadly similar, differences exist between factors predicting primary failure of external cardioversion and recurrence at a later stage. These factors encompass both clinical characteristics and investigational findings.

The answers to these questions allow the physician to decide whether prophylactic treatment is needed, if a regimen for early cardioversion of recurrent AF should be established, whether medical or nonpharmaceutical strategies would be preferred, and if anticoagulation should be considered.

If the patient is in AF, the physician must ask other questions.

- When did the AF start?
- What symptoms does the patient have?
- Has the patient had AF before (if yes, the questions for a patient in sinus rhythm must also be asked)?
- What treatment has already been given to the patient?

From this information the physician must decide whether cardioversion is needed, and if so, when and using which technique. The need for anticoagulation must also be carefully assessed. If it is elected to leave the patient in AF, either permanently or for several days or weeks awaiting cardioversion, the need for and form of rate control must also be considered.

Key references

1. Sopher SM, Camm AJ. Atrial fibrillation: maintenance of sinus rhythm versus rate control. *Am J Cardiol* (1996) **77:** 24A–37A.

2. Waldo A, Pratt C (Eds). A Symposium: Treatment of Atrial Fibrillation in the Era of Managed Care. Supplement to *Am J Cardiol* (1998) **81:** (5A).

Ventricular rate control

9

During sinus rhythm, the discharge frequency of the sinus node controls the heart rate, but in AF the atrioventricular node refractoriness determines the ventricular rate. AF results in atrial depolarizations which probably bombard the AV node between five and ten times a second. Conduction of all or most of these impulses would result in ventricular fibrillation, or haemodynamic compromise. As the ventricular rate rises above 180 bpm the cardiac output reaches a plateau and then begins to fall due to inadequate time for mechanical systole or diastolic filling of the ventricles (the rate for maximal cardiac output is also influenced by other factors such as venous pressure, and systemic vascular resistance). It is therefore important that only a proportion of the atrial depolarizations are conducted to the ventricle. The refractory period of the AV node determines the minimum time between conducted impulses. Its value varies between patients and is very dependent upon the prevailing autonomic tone. An untreated, resting patient with AF will typically have a refractory period of about 500 ms at rest, allowing a ventricular rate of 120 bpm. When the sympathetic nervous system is predominant, during exercise, anxiety, or when AF first begins, the AV refractoriness falls to below 375 ms,

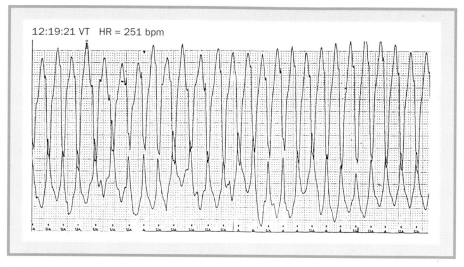

12:19:21 VT   HR = 251 bpm

Figure 32
Holter ECG during paroxysmal AF showing ventricular rates ranging from 150 to nearly 300 bpm despite drug therapy. The broad complex beats are due to aberrant conduction; ventricular tachycardia and an accessory pathway were excluded at electrophysiological study. Such patients are at risk of tachycardia induced ventricular tachycardia, and are candidates for nonpharmacological strategies discussed later in this chapter.

giving ventricular rates of 160 bpm or faster (Figure 32).

There are two important situations where the AV nodal refractoriness does not determine the ventricular response rate: patients with WPW syndrome and dual chamber pacemaker patients. In patients with an accessory pathway (as in the WPW syndrome), the accessory connection from the atrium to the ventricle often has a shorter refractory period than the AV node. During AF, high ventricular rates can occur, resulting in anything from severe palpitations with haemodynamic compromise to haemodymamic collapse or even sudden death (Figure 33). Drugs acting on the AV node, such as digoxin, verapamil and adenosine, will not slow conduction across the accessory pathway and can result in a faster ventricular rate due to improved conduction (either shortening of the accessory pathway refractory period or abolition of concealed retrograde conduction into the accessory pathway), a

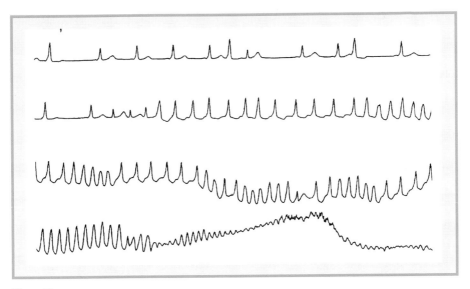

Figure 33
'Pre-excited AF' progressing to VF. This patient had an accessory pathway connecting the atrium to the ventricle. The refractory period of the pathway was short, causing rapid ventricular rates (conduction time is also rapid, but this does not determine ventricular rate). The tracing shows an atrial ectopic initiating regular tachycardia which degenerates to AF with rapid ventricular rates, which further degenerates into ventricular fibrillation. This diagnosis is the most important differential of a rapid irregular broad complex tachycardia, for the reason shown.

negative inotropic effect or vasodilatation. The treatment of choice is to slow conduction over the bypass tract using a drug such as intravenous procainamide or flecainide, or to restore sinus rhythm by urgent DC cardioversion.

If patients with a conventional dual chamber pacemaker suffer AF, the pacemaker may detect the fast atrial rate and pace the ventricle at near its programmed upper rate limit (usually between 120 and 150 bpm). AV nodal blocking drugs will not slow the rate. Instead either restoration of sinus rhythm or reprogramming to a mode which will not 'track' atrial events is required and modern complex pacemakers are able to mode-switch automatically. In response to physiologically inappropriate rates the pacemaker can reprogramme itself to a nontracking mode

('mode switch', for example from DDDR to VVIR) until a physiologically appropriate rate is detected again.

Goals of treatment

Knowing what constitutes adequate ventricular rate control is more difficult than deciding which agent or strategy to use; there are no agreed therapeutic endpoints. It is known that a ventricular rate above 120 bpm for significant periods can reduce the contractility of the left ventricle, and some evidence suggests that harmful effects are present at even lower rates. A ventricular rate at rest in the region of 90 bpm may optimize cardiac performance, but this high rate may have a long-term deleterious effect on ventricular performance. Until more data become available, it seems reasonable to increase the dose of rate limiting medications until tachycardia-related symptoms have been eliminated and the ventricular rate at rest is below 85 bpm. If this cannot be achieved without side-effects, nonpharmacological strategies may be considered, but in asymptomatic cases, serial monitoring of exercise capacity and ventricular function is acceptable. If symptomatic ventricular pauses or bradycardia co-exist with poor rate control, then a ventricular pacemaker combined with rate limiting medications or AV nodal ablation is indicated.

How to assess rate control also merits consideration:

- **Resting ECG or apical rate** should be performed in all cases and is adequate assessment for nonambulant patients (note that the pulse rate may be misleading due to apex–radial deficit; even the apex rate can be unreliable as not all electrical systoles will produce an audible cardiac cycle).

  Goal: resting heart rate = 70–85 bpm.

- **Holter monitoring** is useful for the typical patient with AF. It provides a 24-hour rate profile (it is probably the mean heart rate rather than maximal heart rate which determines risk of tachycardiomyopathy) during normal activity levels, with the ability to correlate symptoms marked in the patient diary with cardiac rhythm.

  Goal: heart rate during activities of daily living (or after a corridor walk/stage 1 of Bruce protocol) < 100 bpm.

- **Formal exercise testing** should be routine in the young and/or active patients. An excessive heart rate response to mild exertion should be avoided while allowing an appropriate response at maximal exercise.

Goal: Bruce protocol stage 1<100 bpm and peak exercise heart rate < (220 *minus* age) for men; (200 *minus* age) for women.

Autonomic provocative manoeuvres (Valsalva, active standing and hand grip) may well provide adequate and cheaper surrogates, but they are not properly evaluated.

Pharmacological rate control

Ventricular rate control in AF can be achieved by direct prolongation of AV nodal refractoriness using non-dihydropyridine calcium channel antagonist drugs such as diltiazem and verapamil. Alternatively, modulation of autonomic influences on AV nodal refractoriness may be employed: digoxin acts largely by increasing vagal tone, and beta blockers reduce sympathetic tone.

At first presentation with AF, the ventricular rate is often high enough to cause haemodynamic compromise and unpleasant symptoms. Restoration of sinus rhythm will return the rate to normal, but if AF has been present for more than 24–48 hours then cardioversion, by whatever means, carries a significant risk of thromboembolism unless the patient is already receiving anticoagulant medications (see Chapter 12). This risk may be accepted if there is severe haemodynamic compromise, but otherwise ventriclar rate control should be instituted. When urgent

ventricular rate control is needed, rapidly acting intravenous beta receptor blocking agents (esmolol) and calcium channel antagonists (diltiazem and verapamil) act within minutes and are strongly preferred to digoxin, which acts slowly (over several hours). Both beta blockers and calcium antagonists are contraindicated in uncontrolled pulmonary oedema or cardiogenic shock, in which circumstances digoxin is often used despite its slow onset of action. Alternatively, the ultra short acting beta blocker esmolol can be cautiously titrated against response where there is concern over adverse haemodynamic effects. Intravenous amiodarone slows the ventricular rate very effectively and is a useful alternative since it is not negatively inotropic. Finally, intravenous magnesium is a quick, safe and efficient method of reducing the ventricular response rate, although seldom sufficient as monotherapy.

When considering long-term therapy it is important to be aware that digoxin does not provide significant ventricular rate control during exercise. There have been a number of small randomized trials comparing digoxin, the calcium channel antagonists diltiazem and verapamil, and beta blocking agents. On balance compared to placebo and digoxin, calcium channel antagonists provide better heart rate control and a small but significant improvement in exercise capacity. Beta blockers do not improve effort tolerance

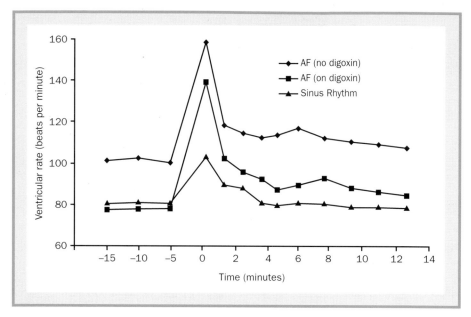

Figure 34
In untreated AF the ventricular rate at rest and during exercise is greater than in sinus rhythm. Following administration of digoxin, the ventricular rate at rest is controlled but that during exercise is unaffected. (Adapted in part from Matsuda M et al. Cardiovasc Res *(1991) 28: 453–7)*

compared to digoxin despite a better rate limiting effect on exertion. Amiodarone is very effective at limiting the ventricular rate, but should be used for this purpose only when other drugs are ineffective.

Verapamil, diltiazem, beta blockers and digoxin are all reasonable as an initial choice for the control of the ventricular rate in AF. The elderly can often be treated adequately with digoxin, or may need no therapy due to poor AV nodal conduction. In younger and active patients, digoxin is very seldom effective as monotherapy due to its poor efficacy at controlling the ventricular rate during exertion (Figure 34). These patients require either digoxin in combination with another agent, or monotherapy with a beta blocker, diltiazem or verapamil (Figure 35). The incidence of side-effects is highest with beta blockers and a calcium antagonist is often preferable in lone AF. Beta blockers have been

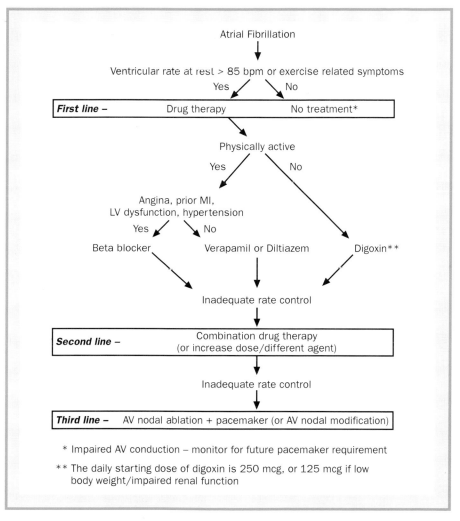

Figure 35
An approach to chronic ventricular rate control in AF.

Table 9
Benefits and drawbacks of strategies for ventricular rate control in permanent AF.

	Resting heart rate	Ventricular rhythm	Exercise heart rate	Overall symptom benefit/QoL	Cardio-vascular risk*
Digoxin monotherapy	Controlled or bradycardia	Irregular	Not controlled	+	→
Beta blocker ± digoxin	Controlled or bradycardia	Irregular	Controlled	+	↓↓
Rate slowing CCA ± digoxin	Controlled or bradycardia	Irregular	Controlled	+ +	↓
AVN Ablation + VVIR	Controlled	Regular	Controlled	+ + +	↓ (?↑)
AVN modification	Controlled or bradycardia	Irregular	Controlled	+ +	↓

*Rate slowing CCA (calcium channel antagonists), verapamil and diltiazem; AVN, atrioventricular node; VVIR, rate responsive ventricular pacemaker; HR, heart rate. *All treatments (with the exception of digoxin) can reverse tachycardiomyopathy, and beta blockers have been shown to improve prognosis for a range of possible co-existent cardiovascular diseases. A small risk of sudden death exists if ventricular pacing is not initially begun at supra-physiological rates (see text)*

shown to provide prognostic benefit in a range of cardiovascular disorders such as hypertension and postmyocardial infarction, but this has to be weighed against their drawbacks.

Key references

1. Redfors A. The effect of different digoxin doses on subjective symptoms and physical working capacity in patients with atrial fibrillation. *Acta Med Scand* (1971) **190:** 307–20.

2. Lang R, Klein HO, Di Segni E et al. Verapamil improves exercise capacity in chronic atrial fibrillation: double-blind crossover trial. *Am Heart J* (1983) **105:** 820–5.

3. Atwood JE, Sullivan MJ, Forbes SM et al. Effect of beta-adrenergic blockade on exercise performance in patients with chronic atrial fibrillation. *J Am Coll Cardiol* (1987) **10:** 314–20.

Nonpharmacological rate control

In some patients with paroxysmal, persistent or permanent AF, symptoms attributable to a high ventricular rate may persist despite 'best' drug therapy, or such therapy may not be tolerated. In such cases control of the ventricular rate can be established by destroying or damaging conduction through the AV node. This may be achieved by catheter ablation techniques using radiofrequency energy. A catheter is introduced into the heart through the venous system and the tip manipulated to the region of the node which lies in the right atrium in the midseptal region, just above the tricuspid valve annulus. Energy is delivered through the tip of this catheter to heat and destroy the underlying cardiac tissue.

Ablation treatment destroys atrioventricular conduction such that the natural ventricular rhythm is determined by a relatively slow intrinsic junctional pacemaker. However, an implanted pacemaker is almost always required to maintain the ventricular rate. If AF is persistent or permanent a rate-adaptive pacemaker is used with a single lead placed in the right ventricle. The pacemaker is programmed to maintain a minimum ventricular rate and to increase this rate when the patient performs exercise. The pacemaker must have a sensor (accelerometer, minute

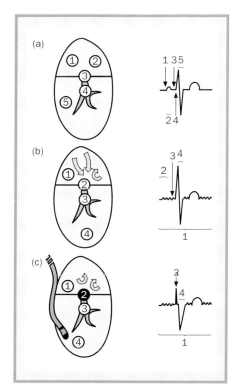

Figure 36
Mechanism of ventricular activation in sinus rhythm, AF and after AV nodal ablation. [a] During sinus rhythm, the cardiac impulse originates in the sinus node (1), activates the atria (2) and the AV node (3). The impulse is conducted slowly through the AV node and then rapidly activates the ventricles (5) via the His–Purkinje system (4). [b] In AF (1), frequent inputs reach the AV node (2), but only a small proportion pass through to reach the His–Purkinje system (3) and hence the ventricle (4). [c] After AV nodal ablation, none of the atrial inputs (1) can enter the AV node (2). It is a stimulus from the pacing wire (4) that activates the ventricles (5). Since activation of the ventricles does not occur via the His–Purkinje system (3), the rate is therefore slower and the QRS complex is broad.

ventilation, vibration, QT interval, etc.) to assess the need for ventricular rate change. If AF is paroxysmal, a dual chamber pacemaker with an additional lead placed in the right atrium must be employed to allow atrial sensing and ventricular pacing during sinus rhythm. Such pacemakers should not track AF, or the patient will experience symptoms due to a high rate of ventricular pacing when in AF. This can be avoided in three ways: the upper pacing rate may be limited (in DDD mode), a nontracking mode (e.g. DDI) may be used, or mode-switching may be employed (Figure 37). A mode-switching pacemaker

automatically changes the mode of pacing from a tracking mode to a nontracking mode when a high atrial rate is sensed, so that the ventricle is paced at the physiologically appropriate rate as determined by the sensor (and reverts back to the tracking mode upon resumption of sinus rhythm).

The use of atrioventricular nodal ablation to control the ventricular rate in AF has been shown to reduce the symptomatic burden in both patients with paroxysmal and persistent AF. Quality of life scores improve, as does exercise tolerance and, especially in patients

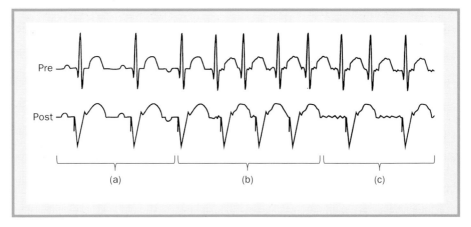

Figure 37
Ventricular rate control during paroxysmal AF by AV nodal ablation and implantation of a mode switching dual chamber pacemaker. Strips (i) and (ii) show the identical sequence of atrial events before and after 'ablate and pace'. Initially there is sinus rhythm (a), and ventricular activation occurs via the AV node (i) or atrial activity is sensed by an atrial pacing wire, which then tracks the signal to the ventricle, which is paced. An atrial ectopic initiates AF (b). Without 'ablate and pace', rapid irregular ventricular activity occurs (i), but with it the pacemaker will not track such rapid activity (ii). After three beats, the pacemaker's algorithm decides that the rhythm is not sinus and switches to a nontracking mode. Thereafter, the ventricle is paced at a regular rate appropriate to the patient's activity level (c) until sinus rhythm resumes.

with a poor ejection fraction, there may be subsequent improvement in left ventricular function. However, it must be remembered that AV ablation is merely a palliative procedure and the thromboembolic risk associated with AF persists. Furthermore, the patient will require a pacemaker for life and could experience syncope or even death in the event of sudden pacemaker failure. Pacemaker implantation increases the probability of progressing from paroxysmal to persistent or permanent AF. This may be because antiarrhythmic agents are often withdrawn following implantation, but definitive data are unavailable.

There is a small but definite incidence of sudden death following AV nodal ablation. This may be due to torsade de pointes provoked by the relative bradycardia following successful ablation. For this reason it is usual to pace at 90 bpm for 1–3 months after the ablation, before gradually reducing the rate to the more normal 60–70 bpm.

It is possible to modify rather than destroy AV nodal conduction, using catheter ablation techniques, to reduce the ventricular rate during AF but a pacemaker is not required. The rhythm remains irregular, and is less efficient than a regular rhythm, but this is counterbalanced by maintaining the more efficient normal ventricular activation sequence. The procedure is attractive, but difficult to achieve in the long term.

Key references

1. Brignole M, Gianfranchi L, Menozzi C et al. Assessment of atrioventricular junction ablation and DDDR mode-switching pacemaker versus pharmacological treatment in patients with severely symptomatic paroxysmal atrial fibrillation: a randomized controlled study. *Circulation* (1997) **96:** 2617–24.

2. Fitzpatrick AP, Kourouyan HD, Siu A et al. Quality of life and outcomes after radiofrequency His-bundle catheter ablation and permanent pacemaker implantation: impact of treatment in paroxysmal and established atrial fibrillation. *Am Heart J* (1996) **131:** 499–507.

3. Kay GN, Bubien RS, Epstein AE, Plumb VJ. Effect of catheter ablation of the atrioventricular junction on quality of life and exercise tolerance in paroxysmal atrial fibrillation. *Am J Cardiol* (1988) **62:** 741–4.

Cardioversion

Pharmacological cardioversion

For the restoration of sinus rhythm in AF patients, DC cardioversion is effective but has drawbacks, such as postcardioversion chest discomfort and the need for general anaesthesia. In contrast, intravenous or oral antiarrhythmic drug administration has few side-effects but requires continuous electrocardiographic monitoring. Once established as safe, however, these drugs can be taken by the patient without recourse to the hospital or physician. Drugs are therefore an attractive treatment modality, but which patients should receive which drug requires careful consideration to avoid inappropriate therapy and proarrhythmic risk.

Drugs in recent onset AF

When approaching the rational therapy of recent onset AF it is important to appreciate that about two-thirds of patients will spontaneously cardiovert within 24 hours. Unless drug therapy trials are placebo controlled a false perception of efficacy may arise, as with digoxin which remains widely used but objectively has an efficacy comparable to placebo.

Several factors influence the probability of pharmacological cardioversion, and these are broadly the same as those already discussed in Chapter 9. Of these the most important is AF duration. Within the first 48 hours following AF onset, cardioversion rates of up to 70% may be expected (Table 10). The efficacy of class 1 antiarrhythmic drugs falls to less than 20% once AF has been present longer, but class 3 agents may remain quite effective. There is little data to support the efficacy of amiodarone, but a number of double-blind trials have been performed using other agents such as sotalol and dofetilide.

Before attempting cardioversion, the patient should be fully assessed to establish any cause for the AF and to evaluate co-existing cardiac disease or electrolyte disturbance. Minimal investigations should include serum electrolytes, 12-lead ECG, chest X-ray and echocardiography except in cases of haemodynamic collapse (where urgent electrical cardioversion is the safer option). The duration of AF should be ascertained, and if doubt exists, cardioversion should be deferred rather than risk thromboembolism. Performing these investigations usually takes an hour or so, and during this time the patient should receive intravenous heparin (5,000 U bolus and infusion of 1,000–1,500 U/hr

adjusted according to APTT/KCCT, or LMW heparin).

Antiarrhythmic drugs are usually administered by slow intravenous injection under continuous electrocardiographic monitoring, but some can be given orally. Adequate resuscitation facilities should be available because adverse arrhythmic complications may occur (Table 11). Individual subgroups of patients are at higher risk of arrhythmias with certain drugs. However in patients with structurally normal hearts and normal electrolytes the risk of an adverse event is low.

Class 1 agents (flecainide, propafenone, quinidine) are effective, while drugs acting predominantly on the AV node, for example digoxin and diltiazem, are ineffective. Amiodarone, sotalol and pure beta blockers have limited efficacy for acute AF but do slow the ventricular rate. Class 3 agents have a much superior efficacy to class 1 drugs for cardioversion of atrial flutter and are also effective for AF. Several new antiarrhythmic agents from this group with significant potential in AF are under development. Dofetilide is orally active, and has been shown to have a neutral effect on mortality in patients with left ventricular dysfunction. Ibutilide is a new short-acting intravenous agent which provides a convenient alternative to electrical cardioversion with moderate efficacy for AF, and high efficacy for flutter.

Table 10
Drugs for cardioversion of recent onset AF (less than 48 hrs duration). Predicted cardioversion rate at 1 hour.

Drug	Route	Efficacy	Comments
Placebo	N/A	+	Without treatment, 15% of recent-onset AF reverts to sinus rhythm at 1 hour, and 60% at 24 hours.
Flecainide	IV	++++	A risk of proarrhythmia exists, as it does with propafenone, quinidine, disopyramide, and to a lesser degree, all drugs. Administering clinician should be aware of the risks, and continuous ECG monitoring and resuscitation equipment must be available.
Propafenone	IV or oral	++++	Cardioversion occurs much earlier with intravenous therapy, but number in sinus rhythm at 24 hours similar for intravenous and oral therapy groups.
Disopyramide, procainamide and quinidine	IV or oral	+++	Rarely used in UK. Disopyramide is effective but causes troublesome anticholinergic side-effects. Procainamide is a first choice agent for AF in WPW syndrome (as are flecainide and propafenone) as it increases the refractoriness of the bypass tract. Quinidine is given orally only.
Esmolol	IV	++	An ultra short-acting beta blocker. Will also provide rate control, but repeated doses or a longer acting agent will be needed in the longer term.
Sotalol, amiodarone	IV	++	These agents provide rate control, lower cardioversion threshold, and reduce early AF recurrence after cardioversion, but are not effective for acute cardioversion alone.
Dofetilide	IV	++	A new class III drug which shows clinical promise, but has not been extensively evaluated yet.
Ibutilide	IV	++	Another new class III drug which is very effective for atrial flutter, but is less effective than flecainide and propafenone for AF.
Digoxin	IV or oral	+	Contrary to popular belief, digoxin is no more effective than placebo at cardioversion. The onset of rate control takes several hours.
Verapamil and diltiazem	IV or oral	+	These agents are ineffective, but do provide rapid rate control.

+ = < 30%; ++ = 31–49%; +++ = >50%

Table 11
Risks from antiarrhythmic drugs.

Bradycardia	*May occur before or, more commonly, after cardioversion. Any agent which suppresses the sinus node or slows conduction in the AV node can cause this (i.e. virtually all antiarrhythmics), and it also occurs after electrical cardioversion.*
Increased ventricular rate	*Some drugs (e.g disopyramide) have anticholinergic effects which can increase AV nodal conduction. Drugs such as verapamil, digoxin and adenosine may result in increased conduction over the accessory pathway in WPW syndrome by complex mechanisms. Alternatively, the fibrillation can be converted to atrial flutter which is rapidly conducted (see figure 49 and accompanying text).*
Hypotension	*All antiarrhythmics are to varying degrees negatively inotropic, and several are vasodilators. In patients with significant haemodynamic compromise, urgent electrical cardioversion or possibly a short acting agent (like esmolol) should be employed.*
Ventricular arrhythmias	*Monomorphic ventricular tachycardia (usually with class 1C agents) or torsade de pointes (with quinidine class 1A and class III agents) may occur. Patients at risk are those with ventricular scarring (class 1C agents), dilatation (class 1A, 1C and III agents), or significant hypertrophy (class III agents).*

Patients with infrequent but long duration paroxysmal AF or with recurrent persistent AF may be suitable for the 'pill in the pocket' approach. This comprises taking up to three standard oral doses of an antiarrhythmic agent over 12 hours when AF episodes occur, with the aim of speeding the return of sinus rhythm. Initial episodes are supervised in hospital, but thereafter the treatment can be taken on an outpatient basis. In general chronic antiarrhythmic therapy is preferred in such patients, but some are intolerant of drugs if taken on a long-term basis. Others find that their drugs do not reduce the frequency of attacks, but do help to terminate episodes. Propafenone has been most widely evaluated in this role, but others can also be employed.

Drugs for long duration AF

Once AF has been present for more than 2 days, antiarrhythmic drugs become much less effective in restoring sinus rhythm. This is probably due to electrical remodelling of the atria by the AF itself, but few data exist to confirm this. There may be a contributory role of other mechanisms such as structural change or autonomic/neural factors.

Although some individual studies have reported higher efficacy, most suggest that antiarrhythmic drugs will only cause about 10% of patients to revert to SR. The one notable exception is amiodarone. In patients who have previously failed cardioversion, a month of oral treatment with amiodarone restores sinus rhythm in between 15 and 30% of cases. It is unclear whether this efficacy reflects class 3 antiarrhythmic action or the other complex effects of the drug. Dofetilide appears to have comparable efficacy to amiodarone from preliminary data, and there are also encouraging results from azimilide.

Other antiarrhythmic drugs have two roles in long duration AF: facilitating cardioversion and preventing AF recurrence, and they have been shown also to affect cardioversion

threshold. In general Vaughan Williams class 1C antiarrhythmic agents (flecainide and propafenone) increase the required energy, class 1A agents (disopyramide, procainamide and quinidine) have a neutral effect, and class 3 drugs (dofetilide, sotalol and probably amiodarone) lower the threshold. The clinical importance of this effect is uncertain. Secondly, prophylactic antiarrhythmics are often commenced prior to cardioversion for practical reasons. A therapeutic serum level of antiarrhythmic agent must be present for the period immediately following cardioversion, when the risk of AF recurrence is highest. Early recurrence of AF (ERAF) is a significant clinical problem for both external and internal cardioversion, and this may be suppressed by antiarrhythmic agents. This benefit may arise by the suppression of ectopic foci that re-initiate AF, but also by altering atrial electrophysiology (increasing the 'wavelet length') to prevent the perpetuation of AF.

Key references

1. Donovan KD, Dobb GJ, Coombs LJ et al. Reversion of recent-onset atrial fibrillation to sinus rhythm by intravenous flecainide. *Am J Cardiol* (1991) **67**: 137–41.

2. Platia EV, Michelson EL, Porterfield JK, Das G. Esmolol versus verapamil in the acute treatment of atrial fibrillation or atrial flutter. *Am J Cardiol* (1989) **63**: 925–9.

3. Gold RL, Haffajee CI, Charos G et al. Amiodarone for refractory atrial fibrillation. *Am J Cardiol* (1986) **57**: 124–7.

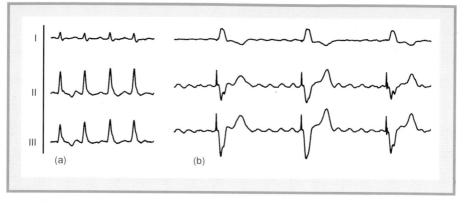

Figure 38
'Ablate and pace' for uncontrolled ventricular response rate in AF: (a) ventricular rate of 140 at rest; (b) the AV node has been ablated and the patient is temporally paced at 60 bpm. When the permanent pacemaker is implanted the ventricular rate is initially set to 90 bpm.

4. The Digitalis in Acute Atrial Fibrillation (DAAF) Trial Group. Intravenous digoxin in acute atrial fibrillation. Results of a randomized, placebo-controlled multicentre trial in 239 patients. *Eur Heart J* (1997) **18:** 649–54.

Electrical cardioversion

The principle of defibrillation is simple: a brief electrical impulse is delivered between two electrode pads, causing simultaneous depolarization of all or most of the myocardium. Automatic pacemaker activity in the sinus node resumes and sinus rhythm is restored. For AF, the defibrillation pads should be positioned to include most of the atrial myocardium within the electric field. The configurations used in practice are apex-sternum (also called 'antero-anterior') and anteroposterior (apex/anterior precardium to below the left scapula, Figure 38). Anteroposterior positioning is associated with a lower mean transthoracic impedance, but has not been shown to be definitively superior in clinical practice. Before accepting that cardioversion is not possible, both paddle positions should be tried. If the shock energy is attenuated by the chest wall (e.g. obese subjects), or by hyperinflated lungs (e.g. emphysema) or if the defibrillation threshold is high (e.g. long duration AF), it may not be possible to restore sinus rhythm.

Table 12
Strategies to effect electrical cardioversion following failure of first shock sequence.

- *Repeat shock at highest energy*
- *Deliver shock at end expiration*
- *Use active compression (i.e. manually applied paddle instead of adhesive electrode pad)*
- *Internal cardioversion*
- *Synchronous use of two defibrillators to deliver greater energy/improved energy field**
- *Use biphasic shock waveform**

* Not currently clinically practised, but the subject of promising research

The success rate for restoration of sinus rhythm by external DC shock is 70–95%, depending on the criteria used to define success and the study population. Success is often defined as a useful clinical result, that is restoration of sinus rhythm for a long enough period to provide some possibility of benefit to the patient. We prefer to make a distinction between failure to restore the patient to sinus rhythm and failure to maintain that rhythm, as these phenomena have quite different implications. A shock which results in sinus rhythm for 5 seconds represents a successful cardioversion but a failure to maintain sinus rhythm and points to a need for rhythm altering medications. With a truly unsuccessful shock, where sinus rhythm is not seen even transiently, it is likely that insufficient energy was delivered to the atria. A range of manoeuvres may be employed to improve the success rate (Table 12) and internal cardioversion may be used if all else fails (Figure 40). Alternatively, pretreating with antiarrhythmic drugs to reduce the defibrillation threshold may be considered. Although this has not been systematically evaluated, there is some evidence to support the use of amiodarone for this purpose.

An electrical shock can initiate as well as terminate fibrillation, and the energy required to initiate fibrillation is less than that required to defibrillate. Initiation of fibrillation is most likely during the repolarization of the myocardium. A shock delivered during ventricular repolarization will often precipitate ventricular fibrillation (Figure 41), whereas a shock which coincides with the QRS complex in sinus rhythm may initiate AF. A low energy shock at any part of the cardiac cycle may

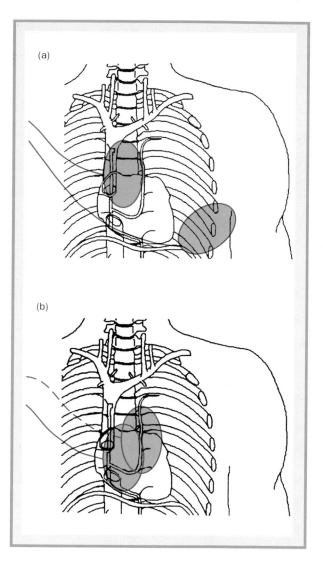

(a)

(b)

Figure 39
The electrode positions used for transthoracic defibrillation.
(a) antero-apical
(b) antero-posterior
(Reproduced with permission from Cardiac Electrophysiology Monitor *(1998) 1: 7–18)*

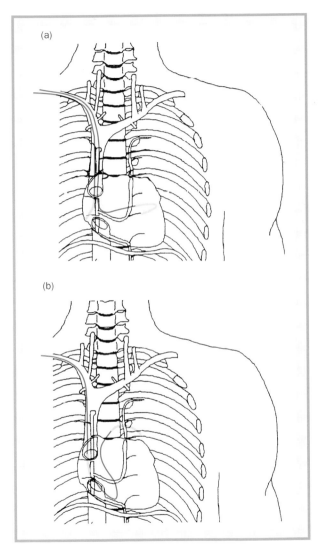

(a)

(b)

Figure 40
Electrode positions used in internal DC cardioversion. (a) shows defibrillation between coils positioned in the coronary sinus and the right atrium. (b) illustrates a 'single-pass' lead. The distal coil is positioned in the left pulmonary artery with the aid of a flotation balloon. The proximal coil is again in the right atrium.
(Reproduced with permission from Cardiac Electrophysiology Monitor *(1998) 1: 7–18)*

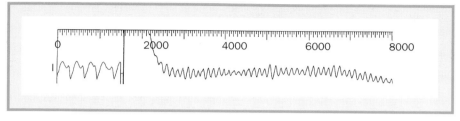

Figure 41
Failure of synchronization. In this case of pre-excited AF, a 50 J DC shock is accidentally delivered during ventricular repolarization instead of synchronized to the R wave. VF results. This was terminated within a few seconds by administration of a 200 J shock.

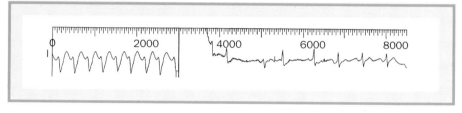

Figure 42
A successful DC cardioversion in the same patient depicted in Figure 41. A correctly synchronized shock terminates AF immediately.

convert atrial flutter to AF. A randomly timed shock has a high probability of falling in the period of ventricular vulnerability, particularly if the ventricular rate is high. By synchronizing the DC shock with a QRS complex, this risk is removed. Accurate synchronization is facilitated by choosing a lead which records a clear QRS deflection but a T wave of low amplitude.

It is usual to first attempt DC cardioversion with low energy shocks. This longstanding policy, endorsed by the American Heart Association, is intended to avoid the use of shocks more intense than absolutely necessary on the grounds that powerful shocks might damage the myocardium. There is no evidence that such damage occurs in clinical practice. The probability of successful termination of chronic AF with a shock of 50–100 J is low and a starting energy of 200 or 360 J is preferred. Initial use of more powerful shocks has the theoretical advantage of minimizing the risk of converting atrial flutter to AF or of initiating VF if the shock is poorly synchronized. Most defibrillators

Table 13
Complications of cardioversion.

Complication	Frequency	Mechanism
Bradycardia/asystole	Common but usually transient and mild. Haemodynamic compromise rare	Due to pre-existing or AF-induced sinus node dysfunction, antiarrhythmic drug use and digoxin
Polymorphic VT	Rare	Thought to be mediated by sudden drop in heart rate, and may also be due to some antiarrhythmic drugs, for example quinidine and solatol
Pulmonary oedema	Rare	Left ventricular dysfunction and neurogenic mechanisms involved
Stroke/thromboembolism	Depends on INR. Very rare if INR adequate (see Chapter 12)	See Chapter 12
Skin burns	Mild soreness not uncommon	Dissipation of electrical energy in the skin. Due to poor skin preparation, faulty electrode pads or inadequate manual pressure

currently in use are incapable of delivering more than 360 J, a level which may be insufficient to terminate chronic AF.

Cardioversion should be performed where resuscitation facilities are available, although problems are very rare in practice (Table 13). A transient bradycardia without haemodynamic compromise is common (Figure 43(a)), but occasionally a profound bradycardia or even a prolonged asystole occurs. Other problems such as acute pulmonary oedema (Figure 43(b)) are also reported. Restoration of sinus rhythm is very occasionally followed by ventricular arrhythmias. With the restoration of sinus rhythm, a sudden drop to slow heart rates can result in polymorphic VT. Quinidine increases the risk of arrhythmia after cardioversion, with a

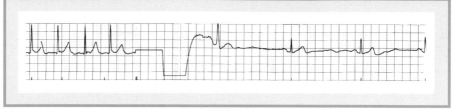

(a)

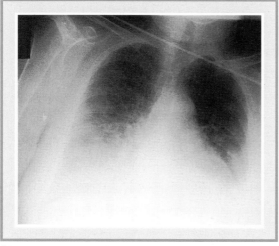

(b)

Figure 43
Complications of cardioversion: (a) a quite marked bradycardia; (b) CXR of a patient who developed pulmonary oedema postcardioversion. The bradycardia was asymptomatic, but the pulmonary oedema was not!

high serum concentration of digoxin being a possible co-factor. It is often recommended that antiarrhythmic drugs and digoxin be withheld for 2 days before cardioversion, but the evidence to support this recommendation is limited and must be weighed against the risk of early AF recurrence if a therapeutic serum level of an antiarrhythmic agent is not present.

A transthoracic shock powerful enough to terminate an arrhythmia is painful for a conscious patient and general anaesthesia or deep sedation with analgesia are required. The source of this pain is predominantly from direct activation of afferent pain nerve fibres, but severe muscle spasm and burning of the skin in direct contact with the defibrillation pads are also involved. Because internal cardioversion requires less energy and because there is no skeletal muscle or skin between the electrodes, the pain involved is less severe. Many patients perceive only discomfort, not pain. Internal cardioversion is therefore usually performed with only light sedation.

Conclusion: complementary strategies

Antiarrhythmic drugs have a valuable role in cardioverting AF, particularly when it is short lived. In appropriate cases such drugs form a valuable alternative to the inconvenience and discomfort of electrical cardioversion (Figure 45). However these agents have a proarrhythmic risk, and it is vital they should not be used without careful patient assessment and the availability of full resuscitation facilities.

Electrical cardioversion is safe and highly effective. However the need for general anaesthesia and other resources, and the inconvenience of the technique, are important drawbacks. Long-term

maintenance of sinus rhythm is poor unless augmented by antiarrhythmic drug use. Finally, internal cardioversion is now available to restore sinus rhythm where external defibrillation is not able to deliver sufficient energy to the atria.

Key references

1. Dalzell GW, Anderson J, Adgey AA. Factors determining success and energy requirements for cardioversion of atrial fibrillation. *Q J Med* (1990) **76:** 903–13.

2. Kerber RE. Transthoracic cardioversion of atrial fibrillation and flutter: standard techniques and new advances. *Am J Cardiol* (1996) **78:** 22–6.

3. Van Gelder IC, Crijns HJ, Van Gilst WH et al. Prediction of uneventful cardioversion and maintenance of sinus rhythm from direct-current cardioversion of chronic atrial fibrillation and flutter. *Am J Cardiol* (1991) **68:** 41 6.

4. Sopher SM, Murgatroyd FDM, Slade AKB et al. Low energy transvenous cardioversion of atrial fibrillation resistant to transthoracic shocks. *Br Heart J* (1996) **75:** 635–8.

Prophylaxis

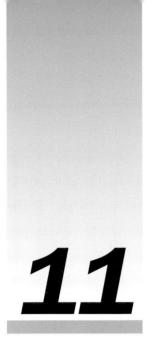

Pharmacological prophylaxis

Antiarrhythmic drugs are currently the mainstay of medical treatment both for the prevention of recurrences of persistent AF and for the reduction of the frequency of episodes of paroxysmal AF. Overall efficacy is only moderate and some patients suffer problems with unpleasant side-effects or more rarely, serious drug-related complications. If used wisely, with regard to both the choice of the patient and the anticipated risks of treatment, these drugs are clinically effective. Injudicious use of antiarrhythmic agents is, however, potentially dangerous.

For untreated patients with persistent AF the risk of recurrence after electrical cardioversion is approximately 50% over the first year. A range of drugs has been shown to reduce the proportion in which recurrence occurs, typically by 50%. Few studies have made direct comparisons between active agents, and placebo-controlled trials are rare so recommendations are based upon inferences from a wide range of data and from clinical practice and experience.

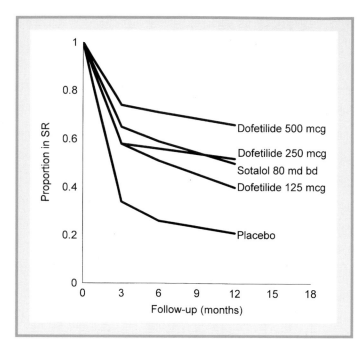

Figure 44
*Efficacy of dofetilide
and sotalol in
maintaining sinus
rhythm post-
cardioversion
compared with placebo
in 535 patients.*
(Greenbaum et al. *Circ*
(1998) 17: 1–663)

Following the first episode of persistent AF, an antiarrhythmic drug is usually not needed. In only half will AF recur within a year, and treating 'all comers' would expose all to the attendant costs, possible side-effects, and potential proarrhythmic risks of treatment. Occasionally, where either the risk of AF recurrence is very high (long duration of AF, ventricular dysfunction, etc.) or where it has caused severe haemodynamic compromise at onset, antiarrhythmic agents are warranted from the start. After a recurrence of AF, antiarrhythmic drug use is indicated except where episodes are infrequent. Once instituted, this therapy should generally be given for at least 1 year. Treatment may be terminated early if side-effects occur, while multiple recurrences warrant long-term treatment. If AF does not recur within 1 year cessation of active antiarrhythmic therapy may be justified, pending further developments.

Choosing which drug to use is an individual decision, and should be based upon familiarity

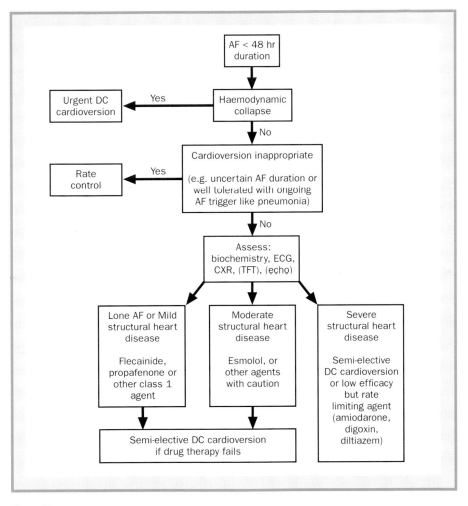

Figure 45
How to approach the management of recent onset AF, and the choice of pharmacological agent or electrical cardioversion.

with a limited range of agents. Our practice is generally to use flecainide, propafenone or sotalol first line (depending on patient characteristics), but all agents have their advocates (Table 14). Because of its serious side-effects amiodarone has a role as a first line agent only for those with significant ventricular dysfunction, but it appears to be highly efficacious. In practice, it is generally well tolerated and the risk of serious side-effects is low if the dose is limited to a maximum of 200 mg daily. As yet there are no good clinical trial data to support the use of amiodarone but most clinicians agree that it is effective and seems to have an appropriate risk : benefit ratio for use in otherwise refractory patients.

Several new class 3 antiarrhythmic drugs have been found to be very effective at terminating and then preventing episodes of AF. Amongst these is dofetilide, which acts almost exclusively by blocking the rapid outward potassium current that is responsible for repolarization of the cell membrane, resulting in prolongation of the myocyte action potential and delayed recovery. It is effective at the atrial level, providing efficacious treatment for atrial flutter and fibrillation, and is largely free of side-effects, except for a 1% incidence of torsade de pointes.

Antiarrhythmic drugs may provide benefit to patients with paroxysmal AF by a wide range of mechanisms (Figure 46). The likelihood of providing a complete cure is very low, but many patients will achieve a worthwhile reduction in the frequency of attacks and significant improvement in their quality of life. It is important to assess the mechanism of symptom reduction. Treatment may alter the pattern of paroxysmal AF from short episodes of rapid AF to long duration well-tolerated episodes due to good rate control. In such a case, the risk of developing persistent AF and thromboembolism may have increased despite symptomatic benefit. The agents used are the same as for persistent AF (Table 14).

In treating paroxysmal AF it is very important to minimize the risk of proarrhythmia. Several of the Vaughan Williams class I drugs (i.e. agents that block the fast inward sodium channel of cardiac myocytes, such as flecainide, quinidine, propafenone, disopyramide and procainamide) may increase the risk of sudden death in patients with myocardial scarring or significant LV dysfunction. While this has been demonstrated only for some agents in the class, all members should probably be avoided or used with caution in at-risk groups. Oral class III drugs (i.e. agents that prolong myocyte repolarization, sotalol, dofetilide and azimilide) and some class I drugs (particularly quinidine) carry a risk of causing torsade de pointes (risk factors are listed in Table 15). Finally class I agents like flecainide, or agents

Table 14

Antiarrhythmic drugs used to prevent recurrence of persistent AF and to treat paroxysmal AF. In paroxysmal AF moricizine, procainamide and cibenzoline have also been used empirically.

Drug	Typical Dose	Notes on dosing	Comments
Flecainide	100 mg bd	Begin at 50 mg bd, maximum dose 150 mg bd. ECG after each dose increase looking for significant QRS widening	Proarrhythmic risks: ventricular arrhythmia (avoid in patients with any ventricular scarring, or with significant ventricular dilatation), 1 : 1 conduction of atrial flutter and exacerbation of sick sinus syndrome. Side-effects infrequent, but if they occur are often CNS related (nausea, dizzyiness, occasional neuropathy).
Sotalol	80 mg bd	Dose range 40–160 mg bd. Below a daily dose of 160 mg may be acting only as a beta blocker	Avoid if significant left ventricular hypertrophy or QT prolongation (risk of torsade de pointes). Monitor QT interval duration. Minor side-effects more common than flecainide and propafenone, **but** the majority of patients tolerate it well.
Propafenone	300 mg bd	150 mg tds, increasing to 300 mg bd. Maximum dose 300 mg tds	Similar proarrhythmic risks as flecainide, but excess mortality in those with structural heart disease remains unproven. Side-effects tend to be gastrointestinal or related to its mild beta-blocking action.
Dofetilide	250 mcg bd	125 to 500 mcg bd. In hospital monitoring for 3 days when commencing	Promising drug but the potential for torsade de pointes is of concern. Avoid in severe structural heart disease and in coadministration with QT prolonging drug. Side effect profile good.
Disopyramide	250 mg bd of SR preparation	250 mg bd (SR preparation), or 100 mg 6 hourly	Effective, especially for those with 'vagal' paroxysmal AF. Troublesome anticholinergic side-effects frequent.
Amiodarone	200 mg od after loading	Load with 200 mg tds for 1 week, then 200 mg bd for 1 week, then 200 mg od. Eventual maintenance dose can be as low as 50 mg od	Moderate efficacy (15–30%) in restoring sinus rhythm in persistent AF without DC cardioversion. Often employed as last resort before nonpharmacological treatments offered, but attractive early choice for the elderly and those with severe structural heart disease. Causes sleep disturbance and photosensitivity frequently, and rarely pulmonary fibrosis.
Beta blockers	Varies	Varies	Little formal testing of efficacy, but reasonable first choice in patients with IHD in whom other agents (except amiodarone) are contraindicated due to proarrhythmic risk. In paroxysmal AF, consider for those with exercise-induced AF or other features suggesting adrenergic onset.
Quinidine	500 mg bd (durules)	250–1000 mg bd (durules)	Not widely used in current European practice, and some concern over proarrhythmic risk causing increased mortality.
Other agents			Treating conditions predisposing to AF (thyroid, chest and heart disease) are helpful both for AF prophylaxis and the patient's general health. Indirect evidence exists that ACE inhibitors, verapamil and diltiazem may reduce the recurrence of AF, but these strategies are currently unproven.

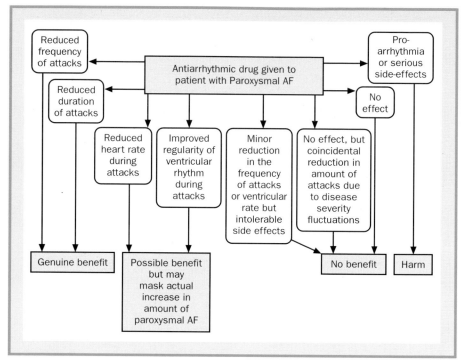

Figure 46
Mechanisms of symptomatic benefit from antiarrhythmic drugs in paroxysmal AF.

such as disopyramide which have an anticholinergic effect, may 'slow' and organize atrial fibrillation into atrial flutter (about 200 bpm instead of the usual 300 bpm), and allow 1:1 conduction to the ventricle (Figure 49). The resultant tachycardia with a ventricular rate of 180–240 bpm often has a wide QRS complex (causing confusion with VT) and may cause severe haemodynamic compromise due to its rapid rate and incoordinate ventricular contraction. The solution is to coadminister an effective AV nodal blocking drug such as a beta blocker or nondihydropyridine calcium channel antagonist. This should be routine for any patient with documented atrial flutter, and seriously considered for all others. This complication does not appear to be as much

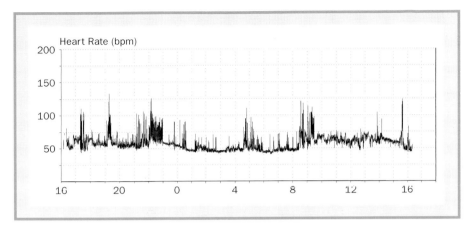

Figure 47
The 24-hour heart rate plot from a patient with paroxysmal AF. Episodes of AF are identifiable as regions with more rapid heart rates and more variability in rate. The accurate automated differentiation of AF from sinus rhythm is very difficult and not currently offered by commercial Holter systems.

Table 15
Risk factors for torsade de pointes during antiarrhythmic therapy.

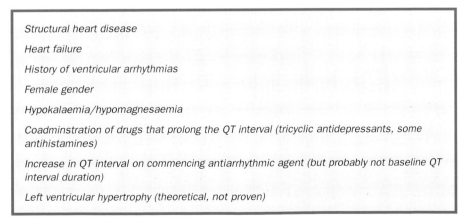

Structural heart disease

Heart failure

History of ventricular arrhythmias

Female gender

Hypokalaemia/hypomagnesaemia

Coadminstration of drugs that prolong the QT interval (tricyclic antidepressants, some antihistamines)

Increase in QT interval on commencing antiarrhythmic agent (but probably not baseline QT interval duration)

Left ventricular hypertrophy (theoretical, not proven)

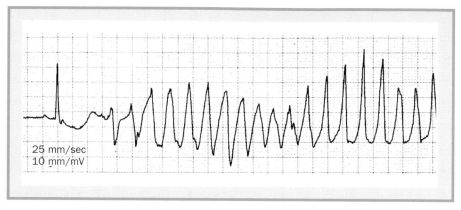

Figure 48

Torsade de pointes. This malignant ventricular tachycardia, characterized by a broad complex tachycardia with sinusoidally varying amplitude, may be induced by several antiarrhythmic agents (for example quinidine, procainamide, sotalol, and occasionally amiodarone). Those most at risk are elderly females, patients with congestive heart failure, anyone in a hypokalaemic state, and those with the congenital long QT syndrome.

of a problem with propafenone, possibly due to its intrinsic antiadrenergic effects.

Digoxin is not effective for the above indications but continues to be widely prescribed. There may be subtle benefits which are clinically apparent without effecting measured variables such as heart rate (see Figure 49) and it has fewer side-effects than most antiarrhythmic drugs. Due to fluctuations in the frequency of paroxysmal AF, therapy initiation can coincide with a spontaneous 'remission phase' and therefore convince both patient and doctor that it is a valuable therapy.

In summary, antiarrhythmic drugs provide a valuable method to prevent recurrent forms of paroxysmal and persistent AF. Many have been shown to be effective, but an individual clinician needs only maintain familiarity with two or three drugs in order to provide good treatment for the majority of patients. Individual response cannot be accurately predicted, and a trial of different agents may be needed before finding the best for a particular patient. Equally, however, the efficacy limitations of drugs should be remembered, and an active policy to switch to nonpharmacological approaches may improve quality of life.

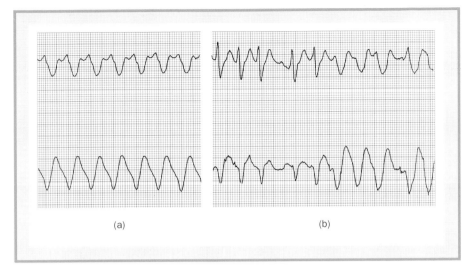

(a)   (b)

Figure 49
Broad complex tachycardia due to atrial flutter, 1:1 AV conduction and functional bundle branch block in a patient with paroxysmal AF treated with flecainide. In (a) a 2-channel Holter recording shows a very broad complex tachycardia which could easily be interpreted as ventricular tachycardia. The true situation is revealed in (b), where narrow complex AF changes to broad complex AF, with the morphology of the broad complexes being identical to during the regular tachycardia.

Key references

1. Crijns HJ, Van Gelder IC, Van Gilst WH et al. Serial antiarrhythmic drug treatment to maintain sinus rhythm after electrical cardioversion for chronic atrial fibrillation or atrial flutter. *Am J Cardiol* (1991) **68:** 335–41.

2. Coumel P, Thomas O, Leenhardt A. Drug therapy for prevention of atrial fibrillation. *Am J Cardiol* (1996) **77:** 3A–9A.

Pacing and implantable atrial defibrillators

The use of pacemakers specifically to prevent AF is a new pacing indication but there are currently few data to support this therapy in unselected patients with AF. However, it is clear that the incidence of AF in patients with a conventional bradycardia indication for pacing may be dramatically reduced by appropriate pacing therapy.

Conventional pacing indications

Paroxysmal AF is common in patients paced for symptomatic sinus node disease, sometimes presenting as the 'brady-tachy' syndrome, and some of these patients develop paroxysmal or persistent AF. Occasionally progressive bradycardia or pauses may be observed just prior to the onset of AF and may be prevented by maintaining the atrial rate with a pacemaker. It is clear that the atria rather than the ventricle must be paced (such that atrioventricular synchrony is maintained). In a prospective randomized study of AAI (i.e. sensing and pacing in the atria) versus VVI (i.e. sensing and pacing in the ventricles), the incidence of AF, cerebrovascular accidents, and death were all significantly lower in the AAI group (Table 16). However, such studies do not indicate that atrial pacing per se prevents AF — the loss of AV synchrony associated with VVI pacing may account for the higher incidence of AF in this group.

Some patients presenting with paroxysmal AF may have subclinical (i.e. asymptomatic) forms of sinus node disease and it is possible that the avoidance of sinus bradycardia in such patients by atrial pacing will prevent the onset of AF. This appears to be particularly true in patients who develop symptomatic sinus node disease only as a result of the antiarrhythmic drug therapy used to prevent paroxysmal AF. The combination of pacing and antiarrhythmic drug therapy may then prevent both symptomatic bradycardia and tachycardia.

Pacing to prevent AF

There is theoretical and clinical evidence to suggest that pacing may be a useful treatment in patients without a conventional indication for pacing. The mechanisms of benefit may be classified into two broad categories.

Table 16
The incidences of AF, stroke and death were lower in the AAI group in a randomized study of patients paced for sinus node disease.

	Number of patients	AF	Thromboembolic events	Death
AAI	110	26	13	39
VVI	115	40	26	57

(Source: Anderson et al. *Lancet* (1997) **350**: 1210–16)

(1) **Preventing bradycardia and suppressing ectopic activity (consistent atrial pacing algorithms).** Preventing bradycardia may be helpful in reducing paroxysmal AF episodes in those with sick sinus syndrome and those with so-called vagal AF. Pacing algorithms that increase in the rate of atrial pacing on sensing of an atrial premature beat or sinus tachycardia are under evaluation. The pacemakers are rate responsive, and some offer rate smoothing, with a 'post-exercise response' which prevents sudden rate drops after exercise finishes. Finally ensuring constant atrial capture by appropriate basal and activity pacemaker rates is probably essential to prevent AF.

(2) **Altering atrial activation.**

(a)   Synchronous pacing of the right and left (via the coronary sinus) atria may be useful in patients with prolonged P waves on the ECG, indicating delayed conduction within and between the atria (which gives rise to electrophysiological and haemodynamic abnormality).

(b)   New site(s) of atrial pacing such as the high and low (coronary sinus os) right atrium, or the interatrial septum alters atrial activation sequence and may suppress AF initiation which might be dependent on specific anatomical patterns of atrial inhomogeneity.

Implantable atrial defibrillators

An implantable atrial defibrillator is not a prophylactic therapy, but is more akin to the 'pill in the pocket' approach with antiarrhythmic drug therapy (see chapter 10). However, clinical evidence is emerging to support the theoretical concept that AF remodels the human atria, and thus reducing the amount of AF will prevent or even reverse remodelling. There are currently two devices. The stand-alone atrioverter is slightly larger than a conventional pacemaker and is implanted in a similar way. A pacing lead is placed in the right ventricle, and defibrillation coils are positioned transvenously in the right atrium and coronary sinus. When symptoms occur, the patient activates the device using a magnet and if AF is confirmed by the device, it will deliver a shock and restore sinus rhythm. Since no facility for ventricular defibrillation exists, avoidance of proarrhythmia is paramount. Numerous measures are incorporated, such as only shocking after an RR interval which is at least 500 ms in duration (avoiding proarrhythmic risk if minor mis-timing of the shock occurs). The device is suitable for those with long duration paroxysmal AF and recurrent persistent AF. The shocks appear to be effective, safe and are well tolerated (some discomfort is experienced but is acceptable to patients given the benefit). The alternative approach is to incorporate atrial defibrillation

Table 17
Who should receive an atrioverter?

Indications for an atrioverter
Recurrent persistent AF or paroxysmal AF with long duration episodes
Resistance or intolerance of standard antiarrhythmic agents*
Desire by physician and patient to maintain sinus rhythm
Patient willingness to accept shock discomfort
Absence of significant structural heart disease and ventricular arrhythmias for stand-alone atrioverter, but this is a relative indication for a dual chamber defibrillator patients with significant structural heart disease may be considered for a combined atrial and ventricular defibrillator
*Antiarrhythmic agents may still be required to reduce episode frequency or prevent AF reinitiating immediately after cardioversion (early recurrence of AF, ERAF) may be used if others fail due to side-effects rather than lack of efficacy. Little trial evidence exists for these agents, but efficacy is expected on theoretical and anecdotal grounds

capabilities into a conventional ventricular defibrillator. Currently one commercial device incorporates a dedicated atrial defibrillation system, but many now offer atrial sensing and pacing, and atrial defibrillation thresholds are higher, but not excessively so, using ventricular coils.

Key references

1. Andersen HR, Neilsen JC, Thomsen PEB et al. Long term follow-up of patients from a randomised trial of atrial versus ventricular pacing for sick sinus syndrome. *Lancet* (1997) **350:** 1210–16.

2. Saksena S, Prakash A, Hill M et al. Prevention of recurrent atrial fibrillation with chronic dual-site right atrial pacing. *J Am Coll Cardiol* (1996) **28:** 687–94.

3. Daubert C, Mabo P, Berder V et al. Permanent dual atrium pacing in major interatrial conduction blocks: a four-year experience. *Pacing Clin Electrophysiol* (1993) **16:** 885.

Surgery and radiofrequency ablation

Cardiac surgery has been used in some specialist centres to prevent AF in patients with very troublesome paroxysmal or persistent AF that has generally proved resistant to other therapies. The operations

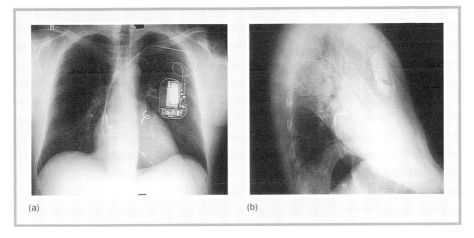

Figure 50
A chest X-ray of a stand-alone atrial defibrillator and lead positions after implantation: (a) chest X-ray;
(b) lateral postero-anterior chest X-ray.

may be classified according to whether sinus rhythm is restored to all parts of the atria such that normal atrial mechanical function and a reduced risk of thromboembolism may be possible, and those which merely intend to restore sinus node activity and conduction to the atrioventricular node.

The operations to prevent AF have been designed following elucidation of the electrophysiological mechanisms which sustain the condition (see Chapter 5). The prevention of AF depends upon interrupting the macro-reentrant circuits that constitute AF. The maze operation involves multiple full thickness incisions across both atria which are then sutured back together creating lines of conduction block within the atria (Figure 51). The areas of atrial tissue between the incisions are not large enough to support re-entry, but the sinus node remains connected to the atrioventricular node and to all parts of the atria by the pathways through the maze enabling it to maintain control of atrial and ventricular depolarization. Such operations have also been applied to patients undergoing cardiac surgery for associated conditions such as mitral valve disease, and have a high success rate in experienced hands. They do however expose patients to the morbidity and mortality associated with cardiac surgery and cardiopulmonary bypass, with particular

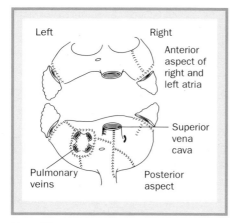

Figure 51
The incisions made during the maze procedure.
(Reproduced with permission from Ann Thorac Surg
(1993) 56: 814–23)

complications including thromboembolism
and sinus node dysfunction. Long-term
cardiac pacing may be necessary.

An alternative surgical approach allows areas
of the atria to continue to fibrillate, but
insulates the sinus node and a tract of tissue
leading to the AV node from these areas by
incisions and cryo-lesions. An example of this
type of operation is the corridor procedure.
These operations have the advantage of
requiring less extensive surgery, but continued
fibrillation, flutter or tachycardia in one or
more parts of the atria means that normal
mechanical function is not wholly restored
and the risk of thromboembolism associated
with atrial tachyarrhythmia persists.

Catheter ablation may also be used to isolate
cardiac tissue by application of radiofrequency
energy which heats the endocardium adjacent
to the catheter tip. Experience with the
catheter maze is limited. The procedures are
long, and are associated with
thromboembolism and pulmonary vein
stenosis following the extensive left atrial
ablation. Linear radiofrequency ablation
techniques are still being investigated. More
limited procedures, within the right atrium
only, carry fewer risks and do reduce the
frequency of AF episodes, but seldom lead to a
clinical cure.

Where there is a documented associated
arrhythmia such as AVRT, AVNRT or atrial
flutter, radiofrequency ablation of that
arrhythmia may cure AF. The results are only
modest, especially in atrial flutter, where AF
recurrences are not infrequent. In patients
who have AF, but administration of an
antiarrhythmic drug converts this to atrial
flutter, the combination of a conventional
'flutter ablation' and continued
administration of the antiarrhythmic agent
can provide a cure. Nonpharmacological
methods may need to be combined with
conventional drug therapies for full benefit.

A proportion of patients with paroxysmal AF
have an underlying atrial tachycardia which
may be eradicated by focal ablation. The
proportion of cases due to this mechanism is

not known but may be high. The clinical characteristics of the subgroup with focal AF are: young, predominantly male, frequent episodes of beats (salvos) of atrial tachycardia which may degenerate into AF, short episodes of rapid AF, and structurally normal hearts (although some evidence suggests that foci may also be important in AF in those with cardiac disease).

Key references

1. Cox JL, Boineau JP, Schuessler RB et al. Successful surgical treatment of atrial fibrillation. Review and clinical update. *JAMA* (1991) **266:** 1976–80.

2. Kobayashi J, Kosakai Y, Isobe F et al. Rationale of the Cox maze procedure for atrial fibrillation during redo mitral valve operations. *J Thorac Cardiovasc Surg* (1996) **112:** 1216–21; discussion 1222.

3. Keane D, Zou L, Ruskin J. Nonpharmacologic therapies for atrial fibrillation. *Am J Cardiol* (1998) **81:** 41C–45C.

Anticoagulation

General principles

Stroke and peripheral thromboembolism account for much of the mortality and serious morbidity associated with AF, and are common in all forms of the condition. Overall, AF accounts for 15–20% of all ischaemic strokes. There is atheroma of the carotid artery or aortic arch in many AF patients, and embolism from this source may account for up to 25% of ischaemic strokes. The incidence of embolic complications during paroxysmal AF is much less well known, but may be up to 2% per annum. Silent cerebral infarction is even more common than stroke. Infarcts may be detected on CT scanning in 15% or more of AF patients without a history of a cerebrovascular event. Silent cerebral infarction would be expected to produce subtle brain damage and it has been suggested as a cause for some of the decline in quality of life, intelligence and memory sometimes associated with longstanding permanent AF.

Prevention with full dose warfarin

In the past decade eight important clinical trials have addressed the prevention of thromboembolism in AF, yielding data which allow calculation of these risks for different patient groups. All of these trials excluded patients with mitral stenosis, or other conventional indications for anticoagulation, as it is generally accepted that these patients have a very high thromboembolic risk and that warfarin should always be prescribed. The trials have been criticized because of low recruitment rates in the screened population, thus impairing wider extrapolation of the findings. Also, target anticoagulation levels varied widely, but were always achieved within the context of a closely monitored clinical trial. It is recognized that such control is often not achieved in clinical practice, and haemorrhagic complications substantially impair quality of life and increase healthcare costs associated with AF. The study population, target INR and outcomes of the five major primary prevention trials for anticoagulation in AF are shown in Figure 52.

The European Atrial Fibrillation Trial (EAFT) was a secondary prevention trial, recruiting patients with AF who had had a TIA or minor ischaemic stroke within the preceding 3 months, with a primary endpoint of death from vascular disease, any stroke, myocardial infarction or systemic embolism.

Oral anticoagulation at a target INR 2.5–4.0 was compared to placebo. In the warfarin group the primary endpoint rate was 8% per annum compared to 17% in the untreated arm (a highly significant difference), and anticoagulation reduced the risk of stroke by about two-thirds.

The efficacy of aspirin and low intensity anticoagulation

Aspirin was compared with warfarin in the SPAF II trial (Stroke Prevention in AF trial II), which found that the risk of stroke was one-third lower on full dose warfarin, but that the rates of major haemorrhagic events were higher. Among patients aged over 75 years haemorrhagic rates on aspirin were 1.6% per year and 4.2% on warfarin, compared with 0.9 and 1.7% respectively in the under 75 years age group. The rates of intracranial haemorrhage in the warfarin group were 1.8% in the over 75 years group and 0.5% in the younger group. In this trial higher degrees of anticoagulation were used compared with the other anticoagulation trials. However, warfarin was especially beneficial versus aspirin in patients with clinical risk factors for thromboembolism (such as a history of a previous thromboembolic event, hypertension or recent heart failure). In Stroke Prevention in Nonrheumatic Atrial Fibrillation (SPINAF) a low dose of warfarin (INR 1.2–1.5) prevented cerebral infarction in 79% of patients without producing an excess risk of major haemorrhage.

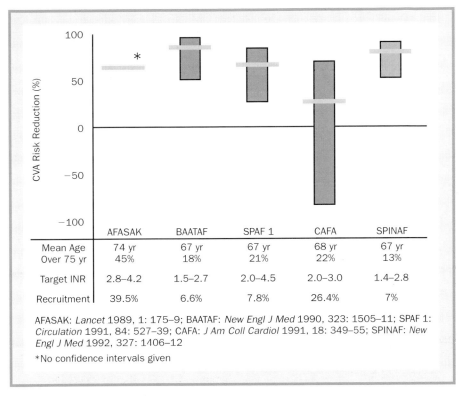

	AFASAK	BAATAF	SPAF 1	CAFA	SPINAF
Mean Age	74 yr	67 yr	67 yr	68 yr	67 yr
Over 75 yr	45%	18%	21%	22%	13%
Target INR	2.8–4.2	1.5–2.7	2.0–4.5	2.0–3.0	1.4–2.8
Recruitment	39.5%	6.6%	7.8%	26.4%	7%

AFASAK: *Lancet* 1989, 1: 175–9; BAATAF: *New Engl J Med* 1990, 323: 1505–11; SPAF 1: *Circulation* 1991, 84: 527–39; CAFA: *J Am Coll Cardiol* 1991, 18: 349–55; SPINAF: *New Engl J Med* 1992, 327: 1406–12

*No confidence intervals given

Figure 52
The effect of anticoagulation with warfarin on stroke in five trials. All of them showed a risk reduction, and this reached statistical significance in all but CAFA, which was stopped prematurely in view of the results from the others. A limitation of these trials is the under-representation of elderly patients, the differing target INR and the often high exclusion rate.

In EAFT patients who could not be anticoagulated were randomized to aspirin (300 mg/day) or placebo. In the aspirin group the overall primary endpoint rate was 15% per annum compared to 19% in the placebo group (a nonsignificant difference), with no evidence of a reduction in the stroke rate (88 with aspirin versus 90 with placebo). Warfarin was compared to 325 mg aspirin in SPAF I and to 75 mg aspirin in AFASAK (Atrial

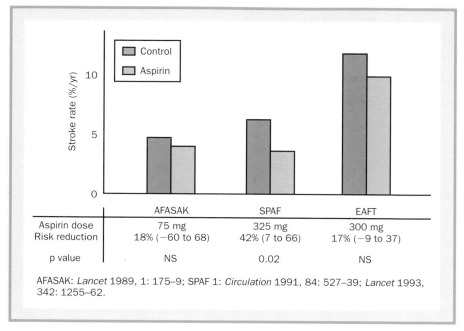

Figure 53
The effect of aspirin on stroke risk in AF in three clinical trials. SPAF is the only trial that showed a statistically significant decrease. Combining these data shows a 21% risk reduction with aspirin (95% CI–37%, p = 0.04).

Fibrillation, ASpirin and AntiKoagulant therapy study). In both cases the event rate on aspirin was lower than on placebo, but the difference was nonsignificant in AFASAK and not as great as the benefit of warfarin in both SPAF and AFASAK (Figure 53).

One trial (SPAF III) compared standard warfarin therapy to a combination of low-dose warfarin and aspirin. Patients in the low-dose arm were given enough warfarin to achieve a

target INR of 1.2–1.5, and then maintained on that dose without further monitoring in combination with aspirin. The trial was stopped prematurely due to significantly higher stroke rates in the low dose arm.

Conclusion

Anticoagulation must be considered in all patients with AF. The decision to anticoagulate is based on an assessment of the

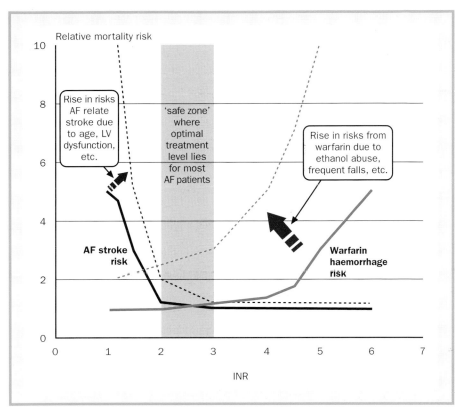

Figure 54
Balancing opposing risks in AF patients. The solid blue and black lines represent the relative mortality risk posed by the AF and warfarin therapy respectively. Each curve may however be pushed 'upwards' (i.e. higher relative risk at any given INR value) by clinical factors, illustrated by the dashed lines. For a patient at very high risk of haemorrhagic complications, the combined risk of treatment and residual AF stroke risk always exceeds the initial stroke risk, and warfarin is therefore not indicated. On the other hand a patient with high AF stroke risk and moderately increased risk of haemorrhage is best treated with warfarin, even though the predicted mortality cannot be returned to age predicted normal.

risk : benefit ratio, derived from all relevant clinical factors pertaining to the risks of stroke and of anticoagulant induced haemorrhage. While the balance is often decided on these criteria alone, echocardiography adds additional independent risk assessment information. Overall AF confers an approximately five-fold increase risk of stroke, and the risk is returned to the age adjusted baseline if the patient is given warfarin sufficient to achieve a target INR of 2–3. In those aged less than 65 years who have no other risk factors such as left ventricular impairment, the absolute annual stroke risk is small (less than the risk attributable to anticoagulation) and anticoagulation is not necessary. In those over 80 years old, few data are available. However the absolute stroke rate is high and the projected benefit is very significant. This must be weighed against the increased risk of haemorrhagic complications and the projected morbidity from such events in the very elderly. Aspirin reduces the stroke rate but is much less effective than warfarin. It may be considered for those at low risk, but the only trial which showed a statistically significant reduction in stroke *used a daily dose of 325 mg.* Data on paroxysmal AF is inadequate, but anticoagulation should be considered if paroxysms are long (>24 hr) or other risk factors such as left atrial dilatation are present. Anticoagulant therapy is definitely indicated if thromboembolism of possible left atrial origin has occurred.

Key references

1. Atrial Fibrillation Investigators. Risk factors for stroke and efficacy of antithrombotic therapy in atrial fibrillation. Analysis of pooled data from five randomized controlled trials. *Arch Intern Med* (1994) **154:** 1449–57.

2. Ezekowitz MD, James KE, Nazarian SM et al.

Silent cerebral infarction in patients with nonrheumatic atrial fibrillation. The Veterans Affairs Stroke Prevention in Nonrheumatic Atrial Fibrillation Investigators. *Circulation* (1995) **92:** 2178–82.

3. Petersen P, Godtfredsen J. Embolic complications in paroxysmal atrial fibrillation. *Stroke* (1986) **17:** 622–6.

Pericardioversion

The risk of thromboembolism is particularly high in the week following conversion to sinus rhythm. This risk may be sharply reduced by anticoagulation, but emboli may occur even if due care is taken. The transient increase in the risk of embolism after the restoration of sinus rhythm is intriguing. There is a widespread belief that the restoration of atrial contractile activity in sinus rhythm displaces thrombi which were formed while the atria were fibrillating. This belief led to an assumption that the absence of atrial thrombus immediately before cardioversion obviated the need for anticoagulation. The assumption proved wrong — a substantial proportion of patients experienced embolic complications despite a normal transoesophageal echocardiograph. Another widely held but probably erroneous belief is that electrical cardioversion causes 'atrial stunning' (i.e. atrial hypocontractility for a period ranging from hours to weeks following cardioversion). Recent evidence suggests it is the preceding AF, not the cardioversion itself, which reduces

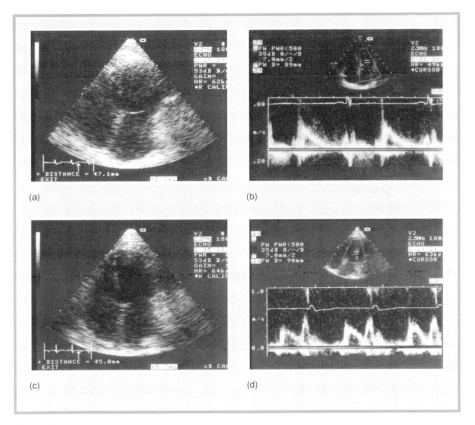

Figure 55
Improvement of left atrial size and function over time following cardioversion. (a) and (b) soon after cardioversion; (c) and (d) 6 weeks later. Left atrial diameter has reduced slightly (from (a) to (c)), and the A wave size increased significantly (from (b) to (d), diastolic Doppler transmitral flow has two components: the E wave, representing passive early ventricular filling; and the A wave, due to active atrial contraction).

atrial contractility. The important practical implication is that the same thromboembolic risk probably exists for pharmacological, and even spontaneous, cardioversion as does for electrical cardioversion. However, the jolt associated with electrical cardioversion could theoretically dislodge left atrial thrombus and result in an embolic complication. Additional effects of DC shock, such as platelet activation, have not been fully elucidated.

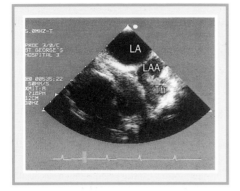

Figure 56
Thrombus in the left atrial appendage revealed by transoesophageal echocardiography. There is a popular but unsubstantiated assumption that thrombi which form during AF are responsible for the emboli which follow conversion to sinus rhythm. LA = left atrium; LAA = left atrial appendage; Th = thrombus.

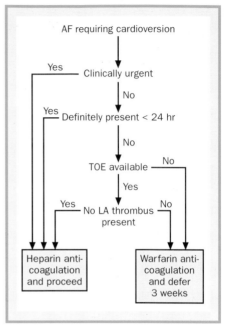

Figure 57
An approach to safe cardioversion of AF. TOE = transoesophageal echocardiography; LA = left atrium. NB. Irrespective of the need for precardioversion anticoagulation, such therapy is needed post cardioversion for up to four weeks.

At least some emboli therefore occur because of thrombus which forms after cardioversion, but whether all are due to this mechanism or whether some are due to pre-existing thrombus is not known. There is no doubt that anticoagulation is necessary at and after DC cardioversion, but whether it is necessary before conversion is unknown. In view of this doubt, the safe course is to follow the established path of anticoagulating all patients for at least 3 weeks before and 4 weeks after cardioversion. The therapeutic INR in this context has not been established. A target of 2–3 is usually recommended but emboli may occur at INRs around 2. It is recommended that a pericardioversion INR target should be 3. This is a better target because fluctuations are less likely to result in inadequate anticoagulation. There is negligible risk from short-term anticoagulation even at higher INRs and embolic complications of elective procedures are highly undesirable.

If a patient presents within 24 hours of the onset of AF, DCC may be performed without prior anticoagulation. Even cases where AF is terminated or spontaneously converts to sinus rhythm within 24 hours of onset, anticoagulation after conversion should be considered as there is a small (0.25–1%) risk of thromboembolism. Although good evidence is lacking, it seems prudent to provide heparin anticoagulation to patients presenting acutely with AF, and to continue it for some hours after restoration of sinus rhythm. Immediate cardioversion is sometimes needed in AF of longer duration if severe haemodynamic compromise is present. Even if it is impossible to anticoagulate before conversion, full anticoagulation for at least 4 weeks after cardioversion is mandatory.

Key reference

Bjerkelund CJ, Orning OM. The efficacy of anticoagulant therapy in preventing embolism related to DC electrical conversion of atrial fibrillation. *Am J Cardiol* (1969) **23:** 208–16.

Conclusions

Active management of AF is important. It is no longer appropriate simply to diagnose the condition and treat the patient with reassurance and digitalis. Many forms of AF can be effectively treated, to such an extent that a cure can be effected in some. The amenable cases are those related to atrial flutter, PSVT, WPW and atrial tachycardia, for all of which the substrate can be ablated and the arrhythmia and the AF it triggers can be entirely or virtually abolished. The role of alcohol as a significant contributory cause of many cases of AF is now more fully appreciated and it is important that, at least at first presentation, a period of complete abstinence should be recommended while trying to suppress any recurrence of the arrhythmia. It is also increasingly clear that it may be crucial to convert AF as soon as it occurs, in order to minimize any electrophysiological and eventually structural changes which will render cardioversion to stable sinus rhythm much less likely. Some focal forms of AF can be identified by Holter monitoring and electrophysiological study, and eradicated by radiofrequency ablation. A large proportion of AF may be due to this mechanism.

Even when AF cannot be cured it may be suppressed by the

Table 18
Appropriate choices of drugs to prevent AF recurrence according to the underlying cardiac disease. Although supported by little efficacy data, digoxin and beta blockers are suggested, based upon safety data and prognostic benefit.
*New Class III antiarrhythmic agents are likely to be adopted as first or second line therapy for several subgroups, but are not currently included due to the paucity of comparative and long term published data.

Cause	First Line*	Next*	Last Resort	Avoid
Idiopathic	Flecainide/Propafanone	Sotalol	Amiodarone	Digoxin
Hypertrophy	Beta Blockade	Flecainide/Propafanone	Amiodarone	Sotalol
Dilatation	Digoxin	Beta Blockade	Amiodarone	Sotalol
Scar	Beta Blockade	Sotalol	Amiodarone	Flecainide/Propafanone
Ischaemia	Beta Blockade	Sotalol	Amiodarone	Flecainide/Propafanone

appropriate choice of antiarrhythmic drug. The challenge is to find an effective drug that will not induce any potentially serious proarrhythmia, more serious than the AF itself. There is an increasingly large number of suitable drugs and the choice can be difficult. Drugs can be eliminated by their potential for toxic effects in large subgroups of patients, thus narrowing the range that is available for any individual. Amiodarone should not be used as first line treatment because of its potential toxicity, particularly when used for long periods. However, it should not be neglected since it is very effective and can be used in low dosages, especially in the elderly, with great success. Drug combinations, especially a sodium channel blocker plus a potassium channel blocker, for example propafenone plus amiodarone, can be very useful. New drugs, such as dofetilide, azimilide and ibutilide are just emerging. The first two appear to have an oral efficacy approaching that of amiodarone but without the complex pharmacodynamics and side effects. Careful monitoring to avoid proarrhythmia (torsade de pointes) will, however, be important.

Repeated cardioversion, atrioversion with an implantable device, atrial pacing and atrial ablation (open-heart surgery, or interventional catheter techniques) offer nondrug-based treatment modalities which are highly successful in appropriate patients. These therapies should not be forgotten, particularly when a patient proves refractory to simple drug therapy.

Therapy for permanent AF is often neglected. However, appropriate rate control is essential and only a small range of drugs is available. The relative inefficacy of digoxin should not be forgotten, but this drug may be successfully employed in combination with calcium antagonists and beta blockers. The potency of amiodarone is also worth remembering in this context although it seldom warrants first or even second line use. It is important to make an assessment of the therapeutic success of rate control strategies; Holter monitoring, exercise testing (formal and informal), and autonomic manoeuvres such as Valsalva, can be easily employed. When rate control proves impossible with drugs, the simple approaches of AV nodal ablation and pacemaker insertion, or AV nodal modification should be considered.

Transoesophageal echocardiography has considerable value in the cardioversion scenario due to its high sensitivity in detecting left atrial thrombus. If there is any doubt regarding the duration of AF, a negative transoesophageal echocardiogram (TOE) provides reassurance that precardioversion anticoagulation can be foregone. However, the need for post cardioversion anticoagulation remains a separate consideration.

The importance of anticoagulation cannot be overemphasized. However, only about 40% of patients are suitable for anticoagulation, and only 40% of these receive anticoagulation. Thus the majority of patients with AF are not effectively anticoagulated and the stroke risk is high in many of these patients. Other strategies to reduce the thromboembolic risk must be considered in such patients. For example, aspirin, good rate control, effective AF suppression and very prompt cardioversion might all be useful in this regard.

In many patients AF is the end result of extensive myocardial damage. In such cases it is unlikely that any clinical strategy will cure AF, but in many others atrial pathology is minimal and associated heart disease is virtually nonexistent. The treatment should be aggressive in such patients and they should not be left to lapse into permanent AF. The retention of good atrial function should minimize thromboembolism, improve haemodynamics, increase exercise tolerance, reduce symptoms and re-establish a good quality of life. The efficacy of AF treatment is rapidly improving and it is very likely that the prevalence of this condition will eventually fall, at least in younger patients. The AF that remains should be treated with close care and attention in order to avoid the serious associated morbidity: heart failure, stroke and sudden death.

Index